Home Chiropractic Handbook

Home Chiropractic Handbook

by
Dr. Karl V. Holmquist
Chiropractor

Library of Congress Catalog Number:
85-62042

ISBN: 0-935081-00-3

First Printing, August 1985
Second Printing, January 1988
Third Printing, March 1990
Fourth Printing, February 1991
Fifth Printing, January 1993
Published by

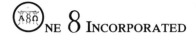
NE 8 INCORPORATED

P.O. Box 2075
Forks, Washington 98331-0822

Publishers Press
Salt Lake City, Utah
Typography by Executype
Salt Lake City, Utah

Dedication

This handbook is dedicated to the principle of the chiropractic philosophy in hope that the people of the world can have better health and happiness through its simple application.

It is written with deep respect for Doctors William and Marion Magiera who practiced chiropractic for twenty-nine years as a husband and wife team. They helped raise from childhood the author of this book. These doctors instilled the highest standard of ethics through living the chiropractic way of life and for their example, the author is forever grateful.

It is written in memory and highest tribute to Doctor Thurman Fleet, a chiropractor and the founder of the Concept-Therapy Philosophy, who demonstrated the principle in its entirety. And in memory of Doctor Charles Craig, a chiropractor who lived life continuing to demonstrate the principle.

Another great chiropractor who without compromise, has remained true to the principle of chiropractic is Dr. Reginald R. Gold. I will always appreciate the inspiration I have received from him.

Special tribute and deep appreciation goes to my wife, E. Renee Holmquist, for her support in thought and action to the principle.

And to my mother whom I've always known to be a fearless lady of iron will.

About the Author

Dr. Holmquist has practiced as a licensed chiropractor in the State of Washington for ten years. He has written this book to advance the knowledge of the chiropractic principle in a way that can literally be brought home to the reader.

Contents

CHAPTER TITLES

Chapter 1
The Purpose of Writing This Book

The primary objective of this book is to provide people with an understanding of how to attain and maintain better health through an understanding of the principle of chiropractic in a way that can be applied in their own homes. Patients of chiropractors and people who have never been to a chiropractor often ask me about the principle of chiropractic and how it actually provides healing benefits. Everyday in my practice I find people telling me how they "popped" their wife's or child's back at home. Many chiropractors are confronted with this situation. Patients comment that they feel better and ask advice. Since people are already attempting to apply chiropractic techniques in their own homes, it has become imperative that they have a basis for proper chiropractic home care.

Being the fourth chiropractor in my family, I have known that every man, woman and child should have their spines checked on a weekly basis. However, this is often not economically possible for the average American family. This handbook insures a medium for cooperation between the doctor of chiropractic and the lay person. The study and application of the principles outlined in this book provide a way for the lay person to accept responsibility in a reasonable manner for his own spinal health and that of his family.

To explain the chiropractic principle, I will refer to *Webster's Dictionary*. The word principle is defined as:

1

la: a comprehensive and fundamental law, doctrine, or assumption b: a rule or code of conduct c: the laws or facts of nature 2a: a primary source.

The word chiropractic as defined by *Webster's Dictionary* is:

a system of healing holding that disease results from a lack of normal nerve function and employing manipulation and specific adjustments of body structures (as the spinal column).

Considering the definitions of these words together, we see that the principle of chiropractic is a comprehensive fundamental law of nature, indicating that disease results from a lack of normal nerve function. The job of a chiropractor is to provide spinal adjustments for correcting and maintaining normal nerve function to release the life energy which flows through the nerve system, allowing healing to occur. More will be said in following chapters concerning life in the body and how it expresses through the body.

This book is not written to teach you to become a professional chiropractor nor to practice chiropractic, nor to diagnose any disease or disease conditions. Rather it is written to help you better understand the principle and techniques, and to assist in home care, thus taking some of the burden off the doctor of chiropractic and to assist him or her in effecting health care. Books have been written on home medical care, and people apply all sorts of medical treatment to themselves. As an analogy, people are technically practicing medicine when they diagnose themselves and prescribe aspirin because aspirin is a drug. Many medical books are now available to the lay person providing at-home suggestions for self-treatment of many health problems. I feel it is time to bring to the public a way to understand and apply the chiropractic principle in correcting the spine at home.

Each chapter that follows has been written in a specific order to fully educate the reader by words, pictures and diagrams. One who diligently studies this text will learn how to detect and correct spinal misalignments. In so doing, you will learn to apply chiropractic techniques so as to attain and maintain better health, consulting your chiropractor when assistance is desired. I suggest the reader take this handbook seriously and make every effort to understand the principle of chiropractic, thereby gaining a deeper understanding of how life flows through your body.

Chapter 2
Chiropractic Philosophy, Science, and Art Explained

To bring the meaning of the title of this chapter into focus, I will again use *Webster's Dictionary* definitions of philosophy, science and art. In chapters that follow, Webster's will also be quoted to help define ideas concerning chiropractic. The reason for this is that the dictionary represents a compilation of what conventional opinion, or mass consciousness has accepted concerning the meaning of words. Words become defined in the context of their use, until a general acceptance of their meaning becomes established. The dictionary then, represents a compilation of words in use and their meaning. More importantly, we can rely on the dictionary to provide us with unbiased definitions, as words are defined in an objective manner. Further, by using Webster's, the reader is granted an objective viewpoint of the philosophy, science, and art of chiropractic and not merely the author's personal opinion regarding what chiropractic is.

Just a side note to the reader: Please read these definitions carefully and do not become dismayed by their use as I intend to tie them together in a 'nutshell' so-to-speak. When I was a little boy, I would look through the "big" dictionary, and my dad, Dr. William R. Magiera, would say to me, "Karl, all you have to do is read that book cover to cover and understand every word and you won't have to go to school anymore." Of course he was joking, but I did gain respect for the amount of knowledge contained in the dictionary.

4

In explaining the philosophy, science and art of chiropractic I will again quote Webster's definition of chiropractic: "a system of healing holding that disease results from a lack of normal nerve function and employing manipulation and specific adjustment of body structures (as the spinal column)."

Webster's definition of philosophy is as follows:

> la: pursuit of wisdom b: a search for truth through logical reasoning rather than factual observation c: an analysis of the grounds of and concepts expressing fundamental beliefs 2a: archaic: physical science (2): Ethics b (1): all learning exclusive of technical precepts and practical arts (2): sciences and liberal arts exclusive of medicine, law, and theology (doctor of--) (3): the 4-year college course of a major seminary c: a discipline comprising logic, aesthetics, ethics, metaphysics and epistemology 3a: a system of philosophical concepts 6: a theory underlying or regarding a sphere of activity or thought 4a: the beliefs, concepts and attitudes of an individual or group 6: calmness of temper and judgment befitting a philosopher.

Webster's definition of science:

> la: possession of knowledge as distinguished from ignorance or misunderstanding b: knowledge attained through study or practice 2a: a department of systematized knowledge as an object of study (the -- of theology) b: something (as a sport or technique) that may be studied or learned like systematized knowledge c: one of natural sciences 3: knowledge covering general truths or the operation of general laws esp. as obtained and tested through scientific method: specif: natural science 4: a system or method based or purporting to be based upon scientific principles.

Webster's definition of art follows:

> la: a skill in performance acquired by experience, study, or observation: knack b: human ingenuity in adapting

5

natural things to man's use 2a: a branch of learning (1): one of the humanities (2) pl: the liberal arts b: archaic: learning scholarship 3a: an occupation requiring knowledge or skill in effecting a desired result 4a: the conscious use of skill, taste, and creative imagination in the production of aesthetic objects; also: works so produced b: the craft of the artist c (1): fine arts (2): one of the fine arts (3): a graphic art 5a: archaic: a skillful plan b: artfulness

The philosophy of chiropractic can be summed up as the pursuit of wisdom or truth using logical reasoning upon concepts regarding the expression of normal nerve function in the body. This logical reasoning dictates a code of ethics through which is developed a discipline to apply the philosophy of chiropractic using the scientific method.

The science of chiropractic can be summed up as possession of knowledge acquired by observation, study and experience; and the application of that knowledge in conjunction with the laws of anatomy and physiology so as to produce normal nerve function in the body.

The art of chiropractic can be summed up as acquisition of the skill required in utilizing the knowledge, and development of a skillful plan or methodology for its application upon the spinal column.

To put the definitions all together: Chiropractic is a philosophy, science, and art dedicated to restoring normal nerve transmission in the body and further, to maintain that normality.

Health in the body is directly related to normal nerve function from brain cell to tissue cell. *Gray's Anatomy,* which is considered a bible of anatomy among the health professions, defines the brain and spinal cord as the central nerve system or the master controlling system. We need only consider who created the human brain, and we know by its magnificent construction that it is the finest computer ever "built." The computer (brain and spinal cord) simply "tells" the body what to do through its 'message trans-mitters' (nerves). The brain is connected to every cell of the body through this intricate message system. To prove this to yourself just wiggle one hair on your arm. This will stimulate that single hair follicle, relaying a message over the nerves, communicating back to your brain. Every cell in every organ of the body is also "told what to do" by the brain through the nerve system. Although you are not conscious of what your internal body parts are doing or even should be doing, the subconscious centers of your brain are sending messages over the nerves and telling every organ and cell what to do and further, coordinating every organ and cell into harmony. Understanding and maintaining this relationship is the key to health through chiropractic. That is, the brain must coordinate messages to every cell (all parts) so that these parts can function normally. If there is interruption in the message due to misaligned vertebrae that put pressure on the spinal cord or spinal nerves, then the body part that receives those nerve messages stops functioning normally and disease may begin to develop.

When you understand the philosophy and apply the science by developing the art of chiropractic, you will have a much better opportunity to enjoy good health and maintain it. As stated in the first chapter, this text must be studied. Although you may never be as experienced or proficient as a professionally trained chiropractor, you can at least begin. Study every chapter deeply and from within; you will develop faith and confidence required to apply the principles of this wonderful philosophy, science, and art called chiropractic.

To conclude this chapter and perhaps lighten up the topic while maintaining its deep meaning, I offer the following statements as conclusive and exact proof of the chiropractic principle.

Many organs and parts of the human body have been removed or replaced by knowledge of modern medical science. People have even lost all four body extremities and yet life goes on in the body, but NO ONE IN THE HISTORY OF MAN HAS DISCONNECTED THE CENTRAL COMPUTER (brain and spinal cord) WITHOUT LOSING LIFE IN THE BODY. In other words, no one has ever had their head cut off and stayed alive. If you can see this truth, you have used your reason correctly and will be filled with enthusiasm in studying this handbook.

Chapter 3
Basic Anatomy of the Spine

Webster's informs us that the word enthusiasm comes from Greek, and means "to be inspired by Theos or God." So dear reader, let's have some fun studying basic anatomy of the spine.

Below is a list of some terminology used in describing the various views of the body and the direction from which you will view them. Memorize these simple terms as they will be of benefit in your study.

Anterior (abbreviated ant.) means front.

Posterior (abbreviated post.) means back.

Superior (abbreviated sup.) means top.

Inferior (abbreviated inf.) means bottom.

Lateral (abbreviated lat.) means side.

A *posterior to anterior view* (P-A view) means looking at it from back to front.

An *anterior to posterior view* (A-P view) means looking at it from front to back.

A *superior to inferior view* (S-I view) means looking at it from top to bottom.

An *inferior to superior* (I-S view) means looking at it from bottom to top.

A *lateral view* means looking at it from the side.

In getting acquainted with the shape of the spine refer to drawing number one in which you are viewing the spine from a posterior view. You can see prongs projecting out on each side, all

drawing # 1

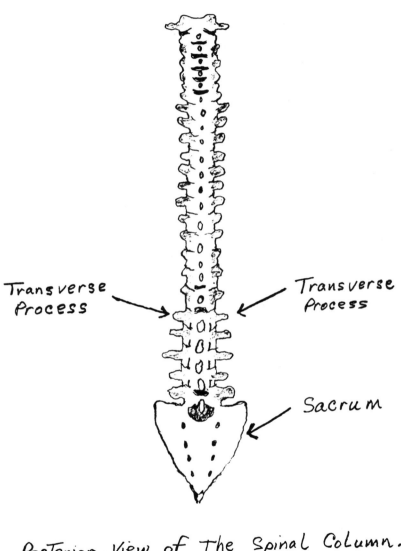

Transverse Process →

Transverse Process ←

Sacrum ←

Posterior View of The Spinal Column.

of various lengths. These are called transverse processes. The sacrum bone fits between the two hip bones to form the pelvis.

The posterior view of the spinal column in Drawing Number 1 is illustrating a straight spine. However, to find a human being with a textbook-straight spine would be difficult. No two people are shaped identical. Just as we all look different on the outside of our bodies, we look and are shaped differently on the inside of our bodies. Each person follows a genetic code and may naturally resemble other family members, yet each member is a unique individual. If you look at your hand and compare it with the hand of anyone else, you will see that it is shaped differently. Your fingers are custom tailored for you. There is not one vertebra in your spine that would fit the spine of anyone else in the entire world of billions of people. Imagine that!

The term scoliosis is a word used by doctors to denote a curvature and the phrase—rotatory scoliosis—means simply a curve with a twist. Now at this point, I would like to make clear some confusing ideas regarding scoliosis. There are just two types of scoliosis:

1. normal scoliosis (normal curve)
2. scoliosis (curve) caused by injury

The second type, scoliosis caused by injury, is rare, as it is the result of some traumatic accident that has actually changed the shape of the spine. This type needs care by a professional chiropractor.

Many times in my practice, patients come in who have been very frightened by some medical doctors and some chiropractic doctors. These patients have been told that they have "curvature of the spine." The technical term—scoliosis—is often used which frightens them. They are often told they will need to wear a back brace for two or three years in order to straighten out the spine. I simply explain to these patients the fact that every human being has a unique shape to his or her body inside and outside. Therefore, there is no cause for alarm.

To further substantiate that every human being has a unique body shape, any doctor can take the same x-ray view of a thousand different individuals and put them on a viewing screen. Not one of

10

these films will superimpose another. Every single film will verify unique curves and contours peculiar to each individual. The unique curves of each individual's spine are genetically designed into the body to balance the person's natural posture and maintain equilibrium. In other words, if the person has a curve in his neck to the right, there will be a compensating curve to the left elsewhere in his spine. Henceforth, the word 'normal' in this handbook will mean 'normal' for you.

This chapter will explain basic anatomy of the spine. The subject will not be covered in great detail; however, it will provide you with enough factual knowledge for later application. It is recommended that the reader supplement his or her study by obtaining a copy of *Gray's Anatomy* or *Grant's Anatomy* from a bookstore or library. Either of these references will afford the student a comprehensive study of human anatomy. If you do take this study seriously, you will marvel at the creation of such a beautiful form as the human body.

Returning to the study of basic anatomy in this handbook, refer to the second drawing of the spine. This is a lateral view. Again let it be clear that the side view of each person's spine is always different than the spine of anyone else. From the lateral view we see people with humped backs, flat backs, flat buttocks, protruding buttocks, straight necks, curved "turtle" necks, long necks, short necks, etc. Virtually all shapes and sizes of people can be observed.

People born with spines that have a peculiar shape such as the humped back individual are often thought to have terrible pain. This again is just an example of variety in life. People having unusual spines may not be suited for normal lifting and sport activities. They can, however, be healthy and free from pain. All that is necessary is for each vertebra to be aligned in conformity with all other vertebrae in their peculiar spine. In this way they can enjoy good spinal health.

On the lateral view of the spine in drawing Number Two, you can see prongs projecting out from the back of each vertebra. These are called spinous processes. Every vertebra has a spinous process except the first vertebra at the top of the spine. The "bumps" you may have felt on someone's back are these spinous processes.

As you can see, the vertebrae on drawing Number Two are numbered. You can also see that the vertebrae on top in the neck are smaller and differently shaped than the ones in the middle of the back. Observe also how different the bottom vertebrae look.

Vertebrae are customarily numbered from the top down. There are seven vertebrae of the neck called cervicals. There are twelve vertebrae of the thorax (mid-back) called thoracics or dorsals. There are five vertebrae of the lower back called lumbars.

The bone that looks like a butterfly from the posterior view is called the sacrum and resembles a hook from the lateral view. Observe the coccyx (tail bone) located at the tip of the sacrum. The sacrum and coccyx are not considered to be vertebrae though they are part of the spine.

drawing # 2

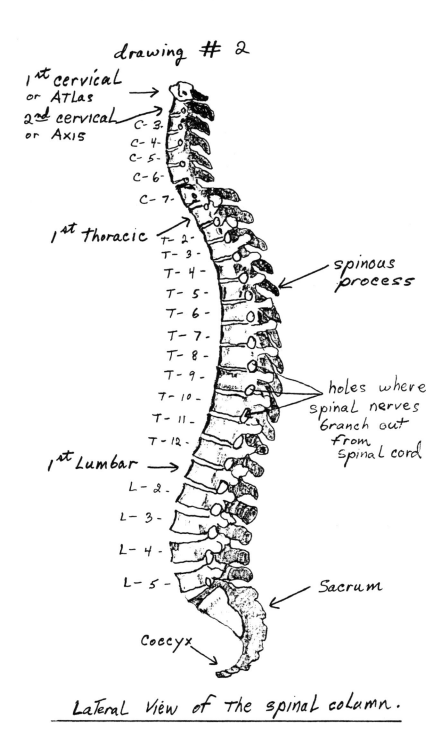

1ˢᵗ cervical
or ATlas
2ⁿᵈ cervical
or Axis

C-3.
C-4.
C-5.
C-6-
C-7.

1ˢᵗ thoracic
T-2.
T-3-
T-4-
T-5-
T-6-
T-7-
T-8-
T-9-
T-10-
T-11-
T-12-

spinous
process

holes where
spinal nerves
branch out
from
spinal cord

1ˢᵗ Lumbar
L-2.
L-3-
L-4-
L-5-

Sacrum

Coccyx

Lateral View of the spinal column.

Drawing Number Three is a bird's-eye view (superior view) of a typical thoracic vertebra. Here you can see the body of the vertebra, the two transverse processes, and the spinous process. Note the pedicles project out from the body and form the superior articular surfaces and underneath form inferior articular surfaces. The lamina on each side is the area between the transverses and spinous. You can also see a foramina (hole or vertebral canal) in the middle of the vertebra. This is where the spinal cord passes down through each vertebra.

drawing # 3

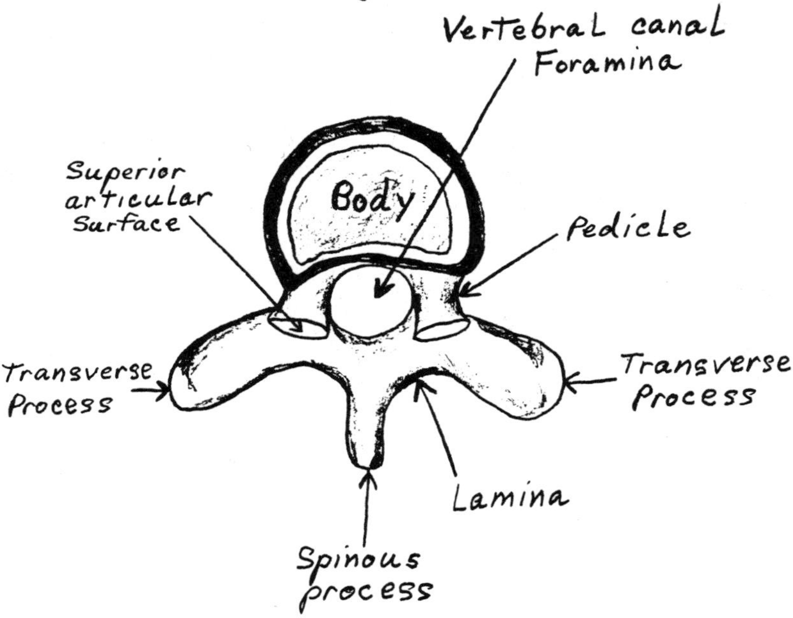

Vertebral canal
Foramina

Superior
articular
Surface

Body

Pedicle

Transverse
Process

Transverse
Process

Lamina

Spinous
process

Superior view of a typical thoracic vertebra

Drawing Number Four is a lateral view of four typical thoracic vertebrae. Note here the holes called intervertebral foramina. These holes indicate where spinal nerves branch off from the spinal cord and go to various parts of the body. There are thirty-one paired spinal nerve roots that branch off and pass through these foramina at every vertebral level. It is through these thirty-one (31) paired spinal nerves that the brain is able to communicate messages to every cell of the body.

A second point to be noted in drawing Number Four are the facets. These indicate where the twelve (12) paired ribs attach to each side of the vertebrae. The ribs form the rib cage. Ribs do not directly attach to the sternum (breast bone) in the front of the body. However, all twelve ribs attach to the thoracic vertebrae in the spine. This is important to understand. A person may injure his ribs and due to the fact that every rib attaches to a thoracic vertebra, the vertebra may be jolted out of normal position or alignment.

drawing # 4

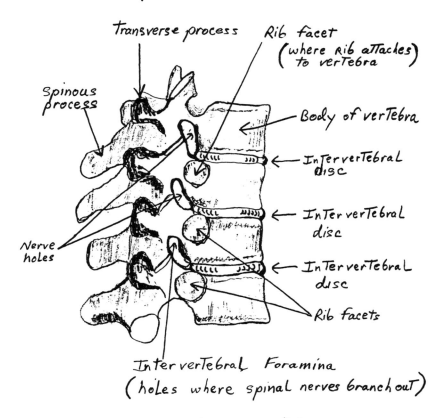

Transverse process

Rib facet
(where Rib attaches)
to verTebra

Spinous
process

Body of verTebra

InTerverTebral
disc

InTerverTebral
disc

InTerverTebral
disc

Nerve
holes

Rib facets

InTerverTebral Foramina
(holes where spinal nerves branch out)

LaTeral View of 4 thoracic verTebrae

Study the next three drawings numbered Five, Six and Seven on the next three pages and note how the ribs attach to the vertebrae.

Drawing Number Five is the complete thorax from a posterior view. Drawing Number Six is the complete thorax from an anterior view. Drawing Number Seven is a lateral view of the thorax.

drawing # 5

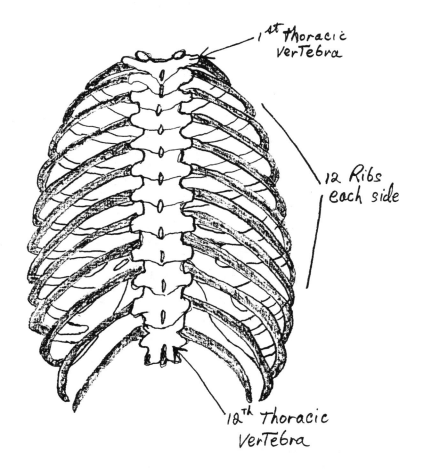

1st thoracic
Vertebra

12 Ribs
each side

12th thoracic
Vertebra

posterior view of complete Thorax

drawing # 6

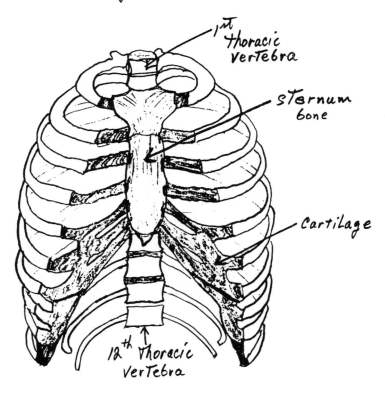

1st Thoracic Vertebra

Sternum bone

Cartilage

12th Thoracic Vertebra

Anterior View of complete Thorax

drawing # 7

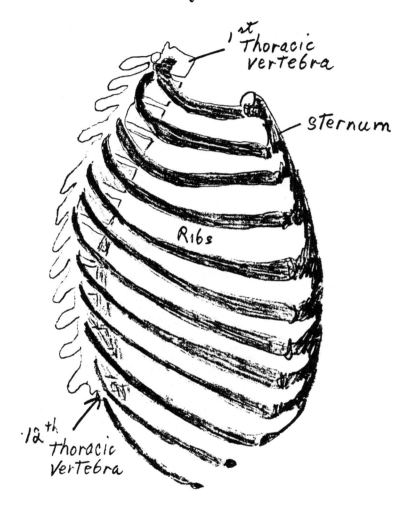

1ˢᵗ Thoracic vertebra

sternum

Ribs

·12ᵗʰ thoracic vertebra

Lateral View of Thorax

21

Drawing Number Eight is a lumbar vertebra seen from a superior view. Study the difference in size and proportions of lumbar vertebrae compared to thoracic and cervical vertebrae. Observe the difference in the shape of the hole where the spinal cord passes down through.

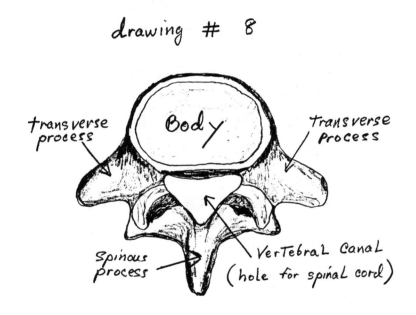

drawing # 8

transverse process

Body

transverse process

Spinous process

VerTebraL CanaL (hole for spinal cord)

Superior view of a typical Lumbar verTebra

Drawing Number Nine is a typical lumbar vertebra. The word typical implies that other vertebrae in a person's spine have the same design.

At this point I would like to state that there are vertebrae considered as *atypical*. In other words these vertebrae are differently designed than any other vertebrae in a person's spine.

Drawings numbered Ten, Eleven, and Twelve offer examples of *atypical* vertebrae. Each of these next three drawings will be considered individually.

drawing # 9

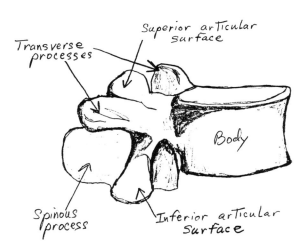

LaTeraL view of a **Typical** Lumbar verTebra

Drawing Number Ten is a posterior view of an *atypical* vertebra, seventh (7th) cervical. C-7 has the longest spinous process in each person's cervical spine relative to all other vertebrae in the cervical spine. This is the vertebra that feels like a "big bump" at the base of the neck. Lamina on cervical vertebra (C-2 through C-7) are projected outward and used for contact points in correcting.

drawing # 10

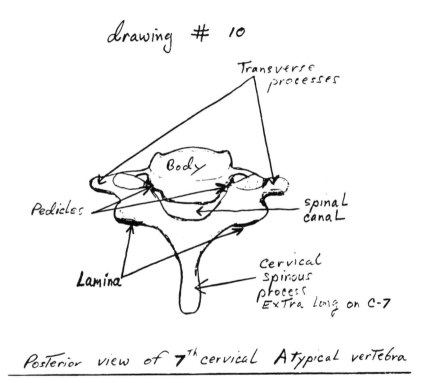

Transverse
processes

Body

Pedicles

spinaL
canaL

Lamina

Cervical
spinous
process
ExTra long on C-7

Posterior view of 7^Th cervical Atypical verTebra

Drawing Number Eleven is the first cervical vertebra. It is *atypical* and has its own name. It is called the *atlas*. As you look at the labeled parts of this vertebra, you will notice that it is very different. It has no body and no spinous process. Instead it is shaped somewhat like a ring and has an anterior arch, a posterior arch, and two lateral masses.

The atlas attaches to the occipital bone at the base of the skull. It attaches below to the second cervical vertebra which is called the axis. There is no intervertebral disc between these two vertebrae. They are held together by ligaments only. Together the atlas and axis can be considered the master key of the spinal column. A misaligned atlas is the only vertebra capable of putting direct pressure on the spinal cord as well as pressure on the branching spinal nerves. Direct pressure on the spinal cord caused by a misaligned atlas can cut nerve transmission (communication) on entire nerve trackways (millions of nerve fibers all at once) resulting in disease in the body.

In chapter five, "Spinal Correcting Techniques Applied," you will be given a simple general correcting technique for the atlas vertebra. However, specific adjustment of the atlas can only be accomplished by a principled, professional chiropractor who utilizes the toggle-recoil method. It would be nearly impossible to explain this method in this handbook.

drawing # 11

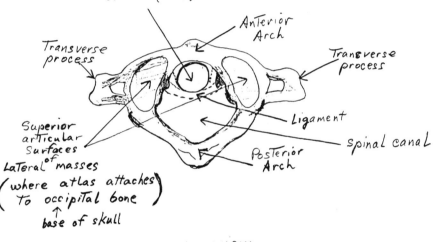

where odonToid process
of C-2 (axis) fiTs

AnTerior
Arch

Transverse
process

Transverse
process

Ligament

Superior
arTicular
surfaces
LaTeral° masses
(where atlas attaches)
To occipital bone
↑
base of skull

Posterior
Arch

spinal canal

superior view
1st cervical verTebra - AtLas - ATypical

Drawing Number Twelve is the second cervical vertebra. It is also *atypical* and has its own name. It is called the *axis*. Make note of the odontoid process of the axis. The atlas vertebra pivots around the odontoid process. The inferior surfaces of the lateral masses of the atlas fit onto the superior articular surfaces of the axis. The normal range of motion must be perfectly maintained in this articulation. (The word *articulation* means joint.)

drawing # 12

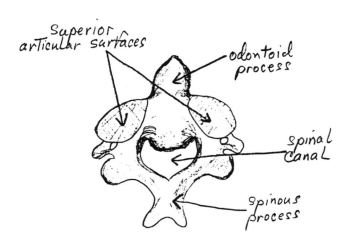

Superior
articular surfaces

odontoid
process

spinal
canal

spinous
process

Superior View
2ⁿᵈ cervical vertebra - AXIS - Atypical

In is now opportune to describe "normal" range of motion. Because every person is built and shaped differently, each person has a different range of motion for his or her articulations (joints). For example, people can be observed who have very muscular builds. They are usually relatively short, stout and powerfully constructed, with thick muscular arms, legs, torso and neck. It can be readily understood that an individual with this type of build would have difficulty in performing extensive stretching exercises. Stretching exercises would not likely hold a natural appeal for the man or woman with a muscular stature.

On the other hand, the individual with a tall, slender build would be more naturally suited for stretching exercises. His or her articulations would respond and move easily due to the inherently flexible and agile stature. However, we can see that heavy weight lifting will never be a serious exercise for this body type as it could be injurious to the articulations.

Understanding the above is the key to enjoying exercise, an important factor when we realize that exercise is required for the maintenance of bodily health. All the individual has to do is select sports or exercises that he or she naturally enjoys and that are in harmony with one's body type.

From the foregoing, you can appreciate that "normal" range of motion for your spine and your entire body is strictly relative to you as an individual. Again, you are unique and differently shaped and thus your entire musculoskeletal system moves with respect to that difference.

Drawing Number Thirteen is a posterior view of the sacrum. Here you can see the articular surfaces where the fifth lumbar vertebra is joined to the sacrum. Observe four foramina on each side of the sacrum where spinal nerves emerge.

In a child the sacrum appears as five individual segments until a mature age at which time the five individual joints fuse and become the one bone called the sacrum.

drawing # 13

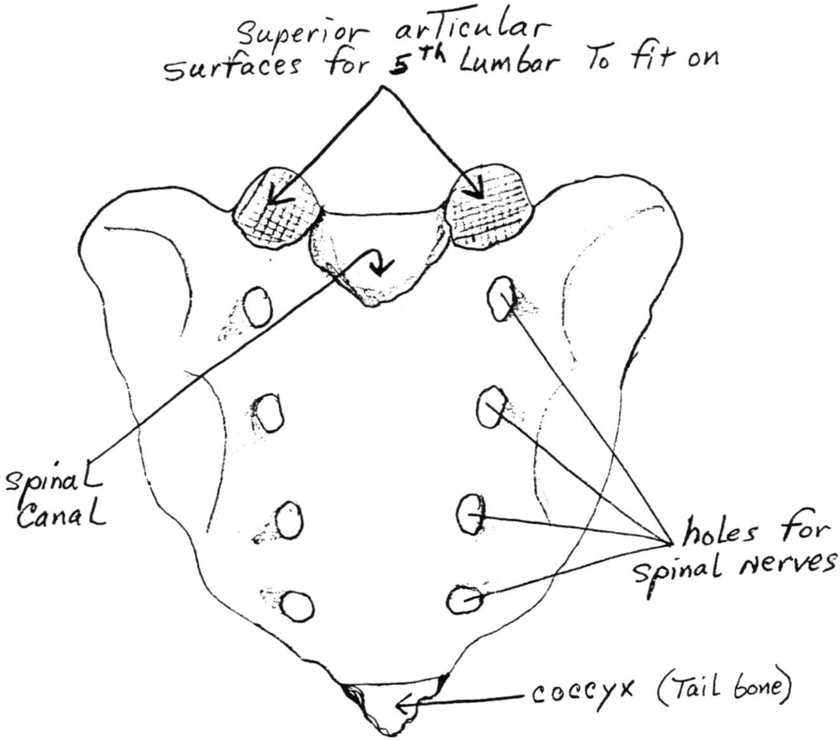

Superior arTicular
surfaces for 5th Lumbar To fit on

spinaL
CanaL

holes for
spinal Nerves

coccyx (Tail bone)

PosTerior view of sacrum

Drawing Number Fourteen is a lateral view of the sacrum and the fifth lumbar vertebra. The one area I bring to your attention is the auricular surface. This is where the innominate (hip) bone articulates with the sacrum.

Also labeled in this drawing is the coccyx (tailbone). People have broken their coccyx sometimes right off the sacrum. Nothing can be done for the patient, except to advise that he use a pillow to sit on. However, the force required to break the coccyx often causes a misalignment of the sacrum and hips, and this will require correcting. The coccyx will not be discussed further simply because no major nerves emerge from the coccyx.

The last feature of this drawing to be noted is where the fifth lumbar vertebra articulates with the sacrum. Here the bottom or last intervertebral disc (sacral base disc) is located between the body of L-5 and the sacrum.

drawing # 14

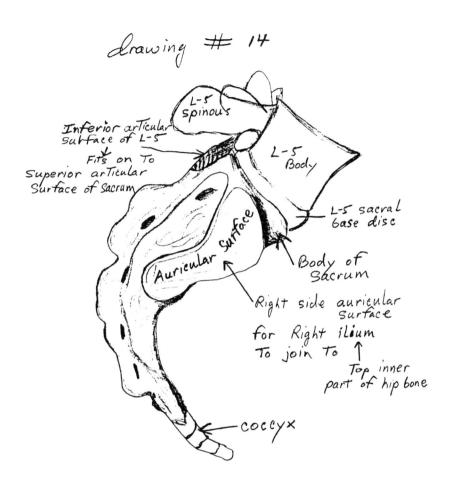

L-5
Spinous

Inferior arTicular
Surface of L-5

Fits on To
Superior arTicular
Surface of Sacrum

L-5
Body

Auricular Surface

L-5 sacral
base disc

Body of
Sacrum

Right side auricular
Surface

for Right ilium
To join To

Top inner
part of hip bone

coccyx

LaTeral View of Sacrum
and 5th Lumbar

Drawing Number Fifteen is an anterior view of the complete pelvis made up of two innominate (hip) bones and the sacrum. Note that *each* hip bone has three parts: the ilium, ischium and pubis. The two iliums articulate with each side of the sacrum on the auricular surfaces. These are movable articulations of the pelvis and must be maintained in a "normal" range of motion. Each hip bone is joined together by a tough ligament. This ligament between the two pubic bones is what softens and stretches through neural and hormonal influence during pregnancy, and causes the pelvis to expand for child delivery.

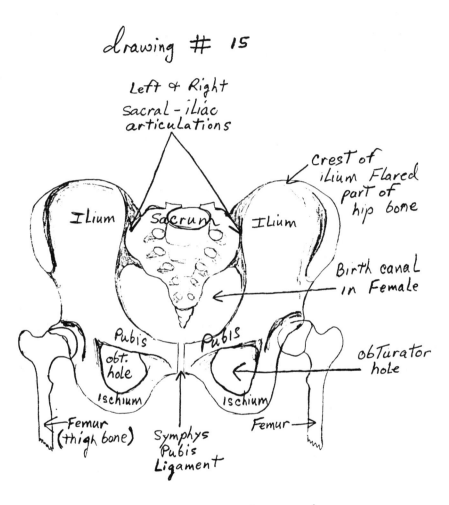

drawing # 15

Left & Right
Sacral - iliac
articulations

crest of
ilium Flared
part of
hip bone

Ilium   Sacrum   Ilium

Birth canal
in Female

Pubis   Pubis

obt.
hole

obTurator
hole

Ischium   Ischium

Femur
(thigh bone)

Symphys
Pubis
Ligament

Femur

Anterior View of complete pelvis

Drawing Number Sixteen provides a lateral view and a superior view of an intervertebral disc. Discs are located between vertebrae from the bottom of C-2 to the base of L-5 and the sacrum. They are made of tough fibro-cartilage arranged in circular fibers as shown in the superior view of this drawing. These circular fibers are called annulus fibrosus. A soft jelly-type material called nucleus pulposus is found in the center of each disc. The primary function of these discs is to absorb shock.

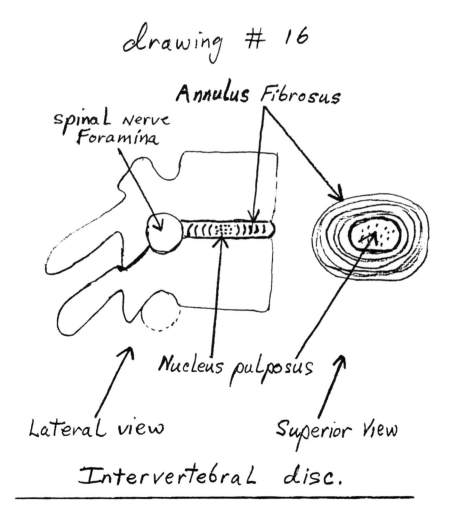

drawing # 16

Annulus Fibrosus

spinaL Nerve
Foramina

Nucleus pulposus

Lateral view   Superior view

Intervertebral disc.

It is now opportune to discuss the intervertebral disc in detail. The term "slipped disc" is a misnomer as the disc does not really move. Discs are firmly attached to the vertebra above and below. In reality what moves is the vertebra upon the disc to a slight degree. In the misalignment of a vertebra, the disc is off-seated, causing uneven pressure to bear upon the disc. This can cause the disc to bulge and *appear* to have "slipped."

A bulging disc is often misdiagnosed as a herniated disc. To clarify this, true herniation of the disc occurs when the nucleus pulposus (soft jelly-like material in the center) ruptures out through the annulus fibrosus (circular fibers) At this point the disc has deteriorated to a great degree.

In cases where the disc is truly herniated the individual experiences very severe pain and is usually directed to have an operation to remove the remaining portion of the disc and fuse the vertebra with the one above and the one below. Therefore, three vertebrae are fused. People with a high tolerance to pain have suffered through this experience, in which case the intelligence in the body heals the area by sending in calcium that naturally fuses the vertebrae. Natural fusions of the spine most often occur in older people, and this causes them to walk, bend, turn their heads, or move in any direction in stiff robot-like movements.

A herniated disc can result from a very abrupt, traumatic accident; however, this is rare. It is most often the result of a misaligned vertebra that has been neglected for a number of years.

It follows, if a person will maintain proper alignment in his spine, these drastic consequences of misaligned vertebrae need never occur. The discs (shock absorbers) will all wear evenly, and the spine will remain comfortable and flexible while aging. The older individual may need to slow down his activities in life, but he can retain health and ease of motion by continuing good spinal care. Furthermore, the opportunity for maintaining health throughout the entire body will be enhanced.

The drawings that follow show how muscles attach to the spine. There are five layers of muscles in the back, forty paired muscles in all. They are arranged and attached in very specific ways to the bones of the spinal column. There are also thirty-three ligaments in the spinal column.

At this point I offer the following terminology that will be helpful for you to know:

> *osteology* — study of bones
> *myology* — study of muscles
> *syndesmology* — study of ligaments
> *neurology* — study of nerves

When studying syndesmology and myology in detail, as all doctors must, every muscle is understood from its exact origin, insertion and action (exactly where and how muscles attach to the bones).

Keep in mind that the presentation of anatomy in this handbook is accurate, but very basic. It is not necessary for the reader to understand all details concerning anatomy. The following drawings numbered seventeen through twenty-three are given to acquaint you with how the muscles appear to attach to the spinal column. For simplicity the drawings will usually show muscles on one side of the spine only. However, spinal muscles are bilateral or paired.

All drawings and schematics in this handbook have been drawn freehand by the author using various anatomy texts for reference. More precise drawings, often in color, can be viewed if you obtain a comprehensive anatomy text, and of course, I highly recommend that you do so.

It should be understood that if the spine is maintained in proper alignment, then the muscles and bones of the spine work in harmony with each other. People often wonder how a pulled muscle affects their back. To answer this question I offer the following example:

A person experiencing a fall or injury can jar a vertebra of the spine out of alignment. The muscles that attach to that vertebra automatically become strained or even torn. Visa-versa, a muscle strained by lifting or pulling too hard, etc., can and most often will pull unevenly on the spine. This causes a misalignment of the vertebrae that the muscle attaches to. People frequently engage in work, sports, and other activities by lifting, pulling, and moving in such a way as to misalign vertebrae. Therefore, it is most advantageous to have the spine corrected on a regular basis. An entire chapter will be devoted to family maintenance correcting of the spine.

The following pages depicting muscles of the spine will proceed without further explanation. Although study of detailed anatomy texts will deepen your appreciation and understanding of the human body, it is not necessary in order to apply the *Home Chiropractic Handbook*. Please observe these drawings carefully and in so doing you will gain an idea of how muscles attach to the spine.

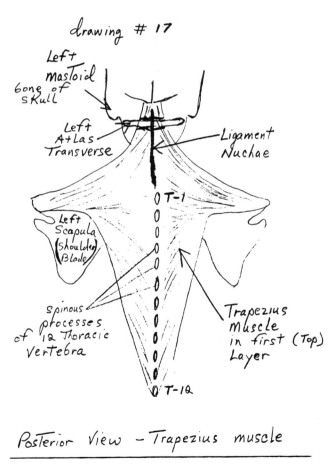

drawing # 17

Left mastoid bone of skull

Left Atlas Transverse

Ligament Nuchae

T-1

Left Scapula (Shoulder Blade)

Spinous processes of 12 Thoracic Vertebra

Trapezius muscle in first (Top) Layer

T-12

Posterior View – Trapezius muscle

39

drawing # 18

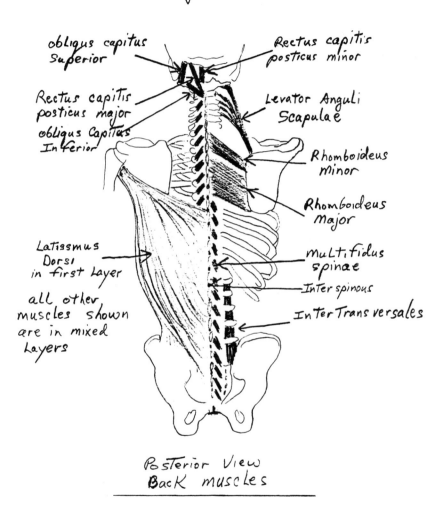

obliqus capitus
Superior

Rectus capitis
posticus minor

Rectus capitis
posticus major

obliqus Capitus
Inferior

Levator Anguli
Scapulae

Rhomboideus
minor

Rhomboideus
Major

Latissmus
Dorsi
in first Layer

all other
muscles shown
are in mixed
Layers

multifidus
spinae

Interspinous

InterTransversales

Posterior View
Back muscles

drawing # 19

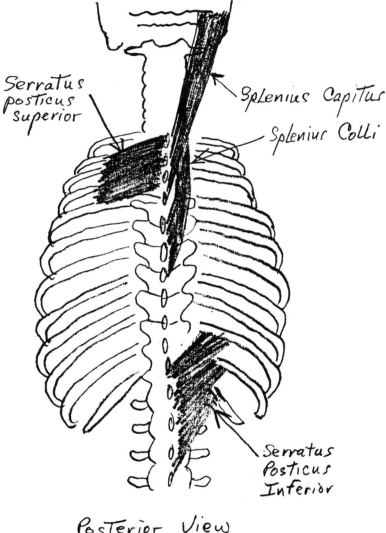

Serratus
posticus
superior

Splenius Capitus

Splenius Colli

Serratus
Posticus
Inferior

Posterior View
Back muscles

drawing # 20

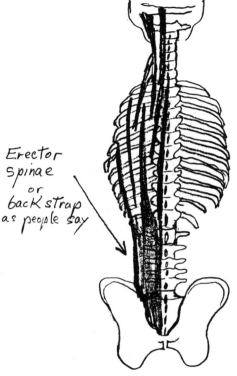

Erector
spinae
or
back strap
as people say

9 muscles comprise the Erector
spinae group further broken
down into 3 of the following
in each Region of the spine
    iliocostalis   - 3
    Longissimus - 3
    spinalis   - 3
        Back muscles
    Posterior view

drawing # 21

Ridges or Lines on base of skull
(occiptal bone) where many muscles attach

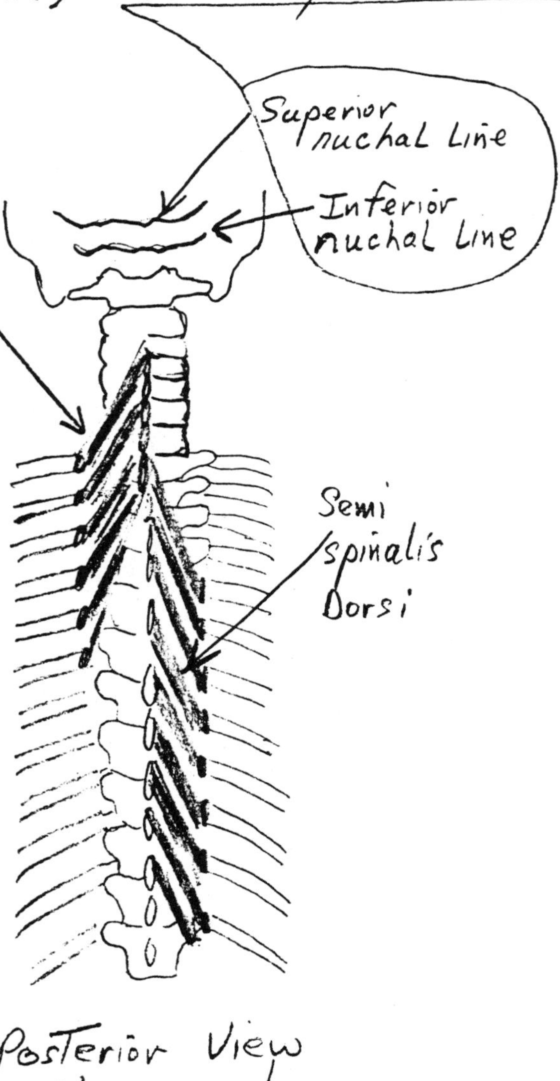

Superior nuchal Line

Inferior nuchal Line

Semi
Spinalis
Colli

Semi
spinalis
Dorsi

Posterior View
Back muscles

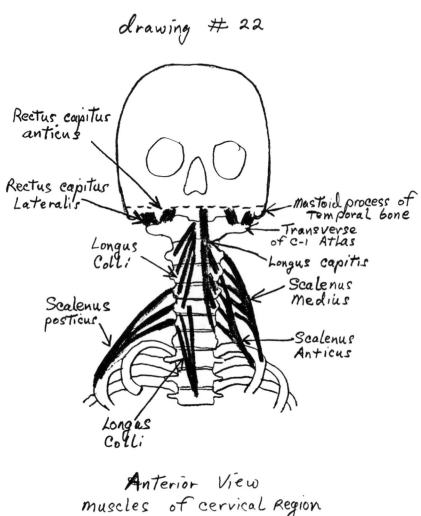

drawing # 22

Rectus capitus anticus

Rectus capitus Lateralis

Longus Colli

Scalenus posticus

Scalenus Medius

Scalenus Anticus

Mastoid process of Temporal bone

Transverse of C-1 Atlas

Longus capitis

Longus Colli

Anterior View
muscles of cervical Region

44

drawing # 23

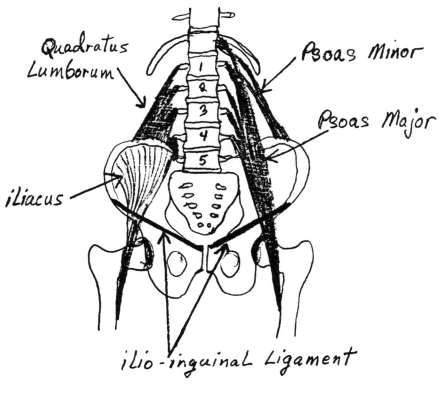

Quadratus
Lumborum

Psoas Minor

Psoas Major

iliacus

ilio-inguinal Ligament

Anterior View
muscles of Lumbar and pelvis

The next portion of this chapter in basic anatomy deals with the six major systems of the body and show how each system is related to the brain and spinal cord. All organs and tissue fall into categories under one or more of these major systems. They are listed as follows:

Glandular system
Eliminative system
Nerve system
Digestive system
Musculoskeletal system
Circulatory system

Every system and each organ within each system is coordinated and regulated by the master controlling system, namely the brain and spinal cord.

Before we continue I offer the following side note. The word *nervous* is an adjective in the dictionary and therefore describes incorrectly the nerve system as being one that is nervous or upset. The body has a nerve system. It does not have a nervous system. When studying the nerve system, you are studying parts of the body under the topic of anatomy. Physiology is the study of the functions of the anatomy or parts. Using the word nervous to describe the nerve system has further suggested to the person that they have a nervous state in their body. This is, of course, undesirable to anyone, and I admonish the writers of anatomy textbooks to correct the misnomer as a suggestion is powerful. I will further elaborate on the power of suggestion in Chapters Nine and Ten.

To give you an idea of just how complex one system is, we shall briefly discuss the nerve system. In studying anatomy, you will discover that within a system there is a system. For example, there is the spinal nerve system consisting of thirty-one paired spinal nerves, and there is a cranial nerve system consisting of twelve paired cranial nerves dropping directly from the cranial vault. These two nerve systems are connected by a sympathetic and parasympathetic system which have the job of speeding up or slowing down nerve impulses between the spinal nerves and cranial nerves. Further, all of these nerve systems are coordinated and regulated by the master system, the brain and spinal cord.

As you can see, the study of the human body is to say the least, very complex. For this reason I intend to show each system in a simple schematic diagram. In these diagrams you will be able to trace the body parts in every system to a specific spinal nerve branching off the spinal cord from a specific vertebral level. By studying the next six schematic diagrams of the major systems, you will gain an understanding of which vertebra to correct in case a particular system or organ is not working well. The foregoing is of paramount importance to you when you consider the fact that a misaligned vertebra impairs the communication of the brain and spinal cord with various end organs resulting in many types of disease. Therefore, vertebral misalignments cause disease as well as pain, disc deterioration and loss of mobility in the spine. However, if vertebrae are properly aligned, they actually protect the spinal cord and insure good health throughout the body.

One last point must be made clear in this chapter. What is a misaligned vertebra and how does it affect the body in a negative way? A misaligned vertebra is technically called a vertebral subluxation. When I consulted *Webster's Dictionary* concerning the word subluxation, it was not specifically listed. Hence, I looked up the prefix sub and the word luxate and found the following definitions:

> sub   1: under, below 3a: less than complete or normal
> 4b: falling nearly in the category of and often adjoining.
>
> luxate dislocated: to throw out of place or out of joint;
> dislocate — luxation.

In combining these we have a subluxation which is less than a complete luxation but still below or not normally adjoining in category (spinal column) and less than in place. The true chiropractic definition describes it more specifically as a vertebra that has lost its normal position and range of motion with the vertebra above and the vertebra below. Ultimately, a subluxated (misaligned) vertebra interferes with normal nerve transmission. It should be distinctly clear at this point that a misaligned vertebra can dras-

47

tically cut down communication of the brain with any body part and thereby cause malfunction and disease.

I suggest you find a library that has a plastic spinal demonstrator or visit a medical library or lab, as you will gain a three-dimensional picture of what a spine actually looks like. This would be of great advantage to your study. Even though each spine is differently shaped, you will glean a good idea of how all the vertebrae fit together.

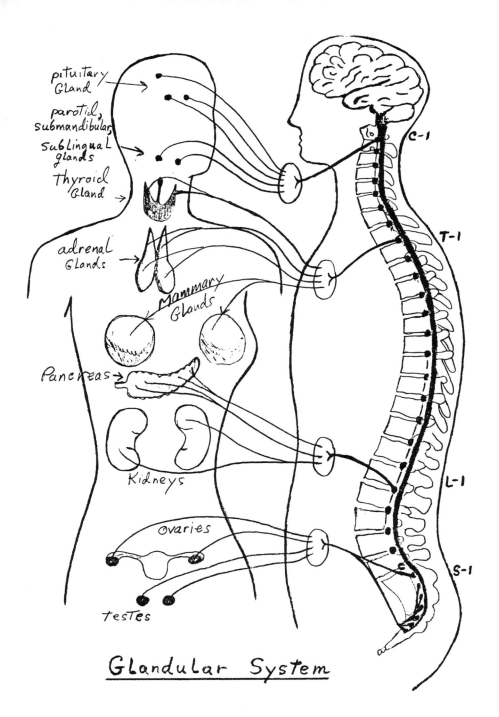

pituitary
Gland

parotid,
submandibular,
sublingual
glands

Thyroid
Gland

adrenal
Glands

Mammary
Glands

Pancreas →

Kidneys

ovaries

testes

C-1

T-1

L-1

S-1

Glandular System

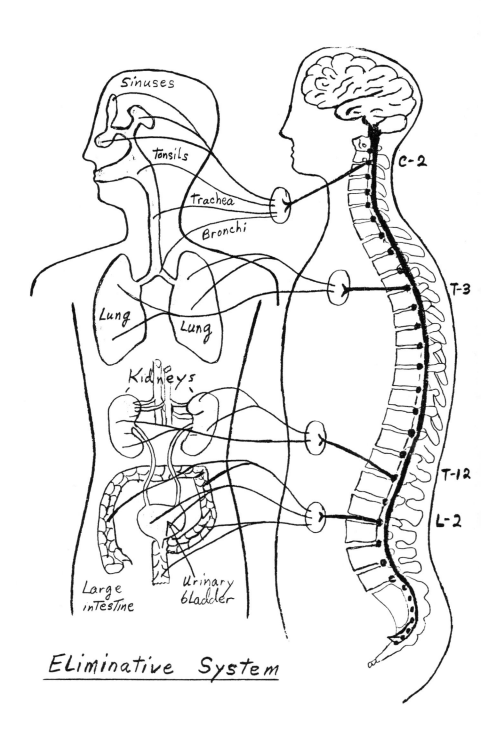

Sinuses

Tonsils

Trachea

Bronchi

Lung

Lung

Kidneys

Large intestine

Urinary bladder

C-2

T-3

T-12

L-2

Eliminative System

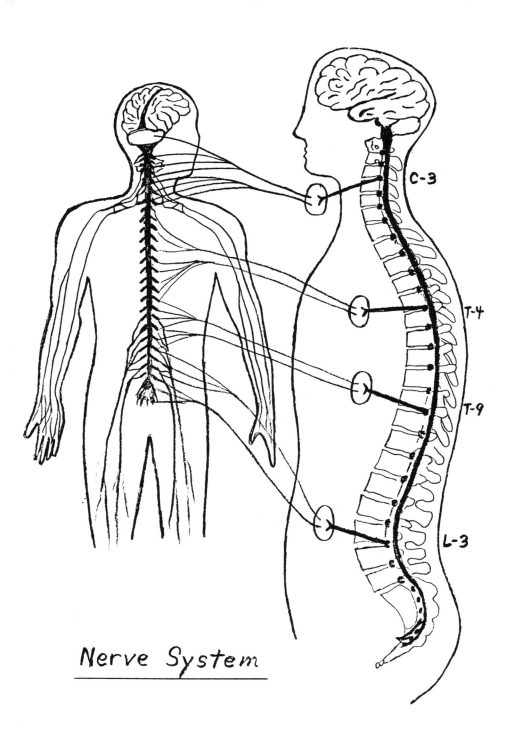

Nerve System

C-3

T-4

T-9

L-3

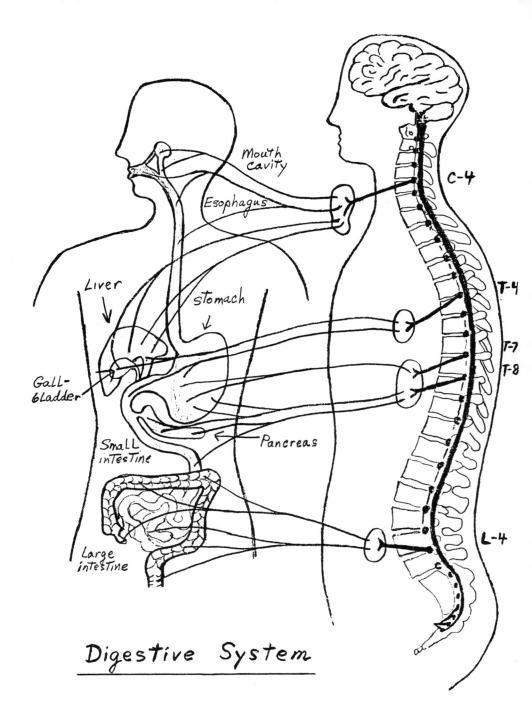

Mouth Cavity

Esophagus

Liver

Stomach

Gall-Bladder

Small Intestine

Pancreas

Large Intestine

C-4

T-4

T-7

T-8

L-4

Digestive System

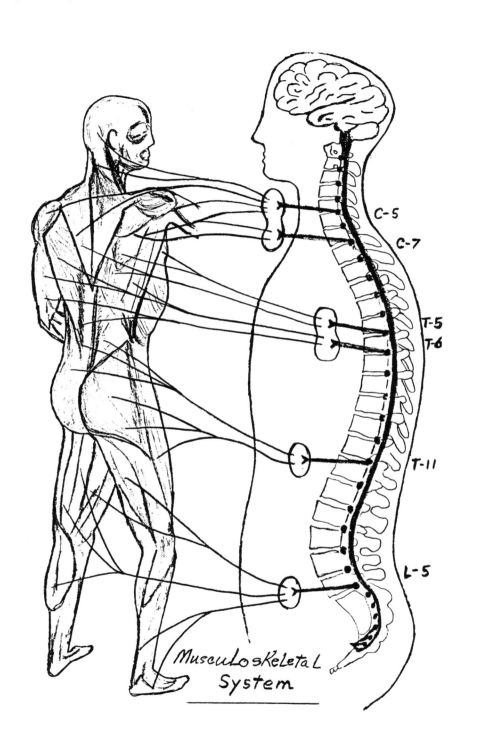

C-5

C-7

T-5

T-6

T-11

L-5

Musculoskeletal
System

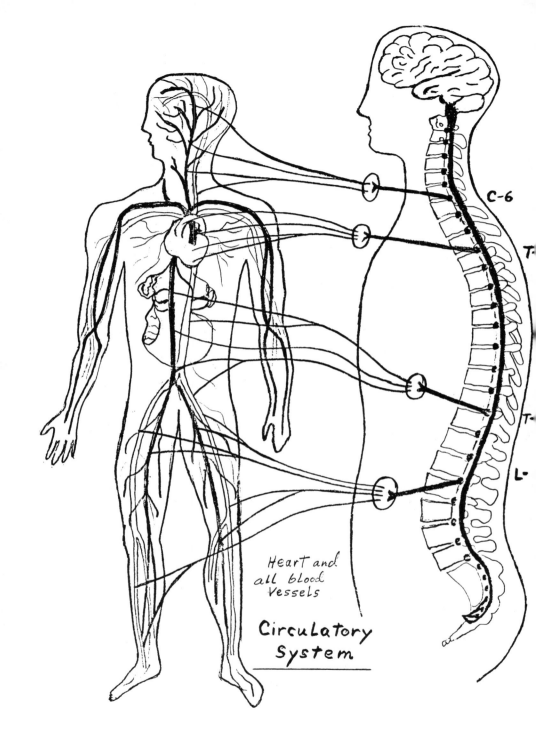

C-6

T-

T-

L-

Heart and
all blood
Vessels

Circulatory
System

54

Chapter 4
Getting Acquainted with Feeling the Spine

The purpose of this chapter is to acquaint the reader with feeling the spine and specifically what he or she is feeling in the spine. Ultimately this knowledge, practically applied, will help the reader to find misaligned vertebrae and correct them.

Again it should be made clear that professional doctors of chiropractic are extensively trained in palpation to locate and give specific adjustments to subluxated vertebrae. Professional chiropractors palpate (the technical word for feel) the spine and locate subluxated (the technical word for misaligned) vertebrae and adjust (the technical word for correct) vertebrae, as needed.

Have a family member wearing a light-weight garment such as a T-shirt or blouse, lie face down on your correcting table. You may use a bed or firm sofa; however, in a later chapter I will show you how to build (or have built) a simple correcting table that will allow a person to lie face down and breathe comfortably through a hole in the table provided for the face. Turning the head to either side on a bed or sofa creates another curve and twists the cervical spine, making it more difficult to accurately feel the thoracic, lumbar and even the pelvic regions of the spine.

Stand at either side of the person to be examined (depending whether you are right or left-handed), and with your fingertips, feel the spinous process C-7, which is the long one in the cervical spine. Just below C-7, feel and count each of the twelve spinous processes of the thoracic spine, T-1 through T-12. Below these feel each lumbar spinous, L-1 through L-5. You may wish to use a pen and actually number each of these by writing the number on the skin over the spinous. In fact, I recommend that you do this. Occasionally, but very rarely, a person is found to have an extra vertebra, perhaps six lumbars or an extra pair of ribs attached to C-7. Follow the above procedure on each member of your family.

Next, spread your first two fingers apart and place them on each side up at C-7 again and slowly move them down along each side of the spinouses. Do this dozens if not hundreds of times. The transverse processes are covered by much muscle tissue and will not be able to be felt nearly as well as the spinouses. *Make note:* you must have read and studied carefully the previous chapter so you can now visualize (hold a mental picture in your mind by concentrating) what the vertebrae look like. You will then be at the *beginning* of knowing what you are feeling.

By repeating the above procedure many times, you may feel that one spinous is off a little to the right or a little to the left in relation to the general shape of the rest of the spinouses. The transverse process will be high (sticking up toward you just a little) on the opposite side of the vertebra. For example, if the spinous of T-6 is off to the right side, the transverse will usually be high on the left side. The spinous processes of the thoracic vertebrae overlap to a great degree. In other words, the spinouses of the thoracic vertebrae are quite a bit longer than spinouses in other areas of the spine. Therefore, they are lower than the transverses of the same vertebrae they are attached to. Apply gentle pressure to the area where you have detected a possible misalignment, and ask the person if he or she feels any tenderness or pain. If he or she says yes, this is a good indication that you have found a misalignment. Remember, pain is always a warning signal sent back to the brain telling the person that something is wrong. It is foolish to cover up pain. By doing so, you are avoiding the problem and not correcting that which is causing the pain. However, do not attempt to make any corrections while studying this chapter.

Before continuing, I would like to inform the reader that every single spinal nerve root contains both sensory and motor nerves. You may not feel any pain in an area of possible misalignment due to the misaligned vertebra putting pressure on the motor portion of the nerve only. In cases where there is no pain, the misaligned vertebra will still disturb normal nerve transmission to the end organ. As an example, a misaligned T-8 vertebra would affect the stomach. One may not feel any tenderness over the spinous or transverses of T-8 and yet may still experience stomach problems due to impaired nerve transmission.

For this reason it is important to check the spine once a week even if there is no spinal pain. If I ask, "What is your liver doing right now?" You would likely answer, "Well, I don't know," and that is true. Even a doctor does not know what his or her own liver is doing at any given moment. The doctor may know all the functions of the liver and where it is located in the body but will never know how to run his or her own liver. Incidently, to further marvel at the human body, scientists tell us the liver has over 350 functions to perform. Could you imagine your conscious brain trying to remember how to keep just your liver functioning? Fortunately, it is all done for you subconsciously and automatically, as long as no misaligned vertebra interferes with the messages from the brain to the liver.

From the foregoing, you now know that there can be a misalignment affecting an organ or body part without pain in the spine. Numbness in the arms, legs, fingers, toes, or other parts of the body also indicates a loss of function of motor nerves. Use your muscular system chart to trace back to misaligned vertebrae that are causing malfunction. But also use your intelligence. For example, if there has been a severe injury to the right elbow, and the right hand is numb, the damage to the nerves would likely be in the elbow and may require attention from a medical doctor.

To continue with the main topic of this chapter—feeling the spine—have the person to be examined lie on his or her stomach. Roll back the person's underwear the bear the skin over the top part of the buttocks. Except for very heavy people you will usually see two dimples on the skin. Place each of your thumbs on those dimples with the remaining fingers of each hand resting on the top of the iliums. These dimples are where the posterior crest of the iliums fit onto the auricular surface of each side of the sacrum.

Apply gentle pressure with your thumbs and ask if there is any tenderness or pain. If the answer is yes on either or both sides, then that individual is suffering from some degree of misalignment. If there is no tenderness or pain but one hip appears high and one low, there may still be a misalignment.

It is appropriate here to sidetrack a little and discuss leg measurement and difference. If I examined one hundred people and measured the length of their legs, at least half of these would not have an equal leg measurement. Now what does this mean? There are two types of leg deficiencies. In the first type the person was born with one of the bones of the leg malformed, causing one leg to be shorter than the other. Due to an injury or break, one leg may be shorter than the other. This first type is called an anatomical leg deficiency. It can be corrected with a heel lift and the exact measurement should be determined by a chiropractor.

The second type of leg deficiency, where the bones of both legs (femurs, tibias, and fibulas) are the same in length yet one leg appears shorter, is due to one hip drawing the leg upward. This type is a physiological or functional deficiency. It is much more common than the first type of leg deficiency and can be corrected by correcting the pelvis or spine. The following check will help you determine whether a pelvic correction is needed:

This leg check is made with the person lying face down. Gently pull both ankles with equal force to straighten the patient's body on the correcting table. It is sometimes best to have the person wear good square-heeled shoes (unworn heels) for this measurement. Now push the shoes together and with your thumbs on the soles of the shoes and fingers around the ankles, equally push upward toward the person's head. If you notice one heel is definitely shorter than the other, it is possible that the hip on that side is high or drawn upward. Make notes on each family member as each individual will usually misalign in the same way due to simple genetic weaknesses in the area.

Part Two of this check requires that both legs be bent at the knees. If the same leg remains short as in Part One of this check, the misalignment is the hip on that side, which has moved anterior and superior (forward and high). If the heels equal out in length or the opposite one becomes the short one, then the misalignment causing it could be anywhere in the spine.

Part Three of this check continues with the person again lying on his or her stomach, face down, legs down (not bent at the knees). Measure the same as in Part One, but ask the person to turn his or her head all the way to the left slowly. If the heels equal out, then the misalignment is in the cervical spine on the side turned down on the table, in this case, the right side. Ask the person to turn his or her head all the way to the right slowly. If the heels equal out, then the misalignment is in the cervical spine on the side of the head that is down on the table, in this case, the left side. The vertebra most often misaligned in these cases, is the Atlas and the third part of this check indicates the side the Atlas has misaligned toward. This will almost always be a constant in each person. Jot down which side each member of your family's atlas lists toward, right or left. The foregoing has been a complete orthopedic check.

In feeling the cervical spine, begin by having the person lie on his or her back and straighten the body out gently. Place both hands on each side of the neck and with the fingers of each hand, beginning at C-7, move up feeling the spinous processes. Remember C-1, the Atlas, has no spinous and cannot be felt from the back of the neck. Count all six of the remaining processes of the cervical spine. Do this many, many times. Now go back to C-7, somewhat cradling the head in both of your hands and feel the transverses which are very short. Nearly every transverse can be sensitive to the person as you feel them and should never be contacted to make a correction. Feeling between the spinouses and transverses, you will find the lamina (refer to drawing number 10) in Chapter Three, to help visualize the lamina). Lamina should be felt on each vertebra from C-7 up to C-2. Here is where one side may feel more tender or painful than the other side. Feel these over and over again, picturing in your mind what you are feeling, while recalling your study of anatomy. Although no pain is expressed upon questioning the person, one side may be off and rotated. If the spinous of a cervical vertebra is off to one side, the lamina will be rotated to the opposite side. Without detailed study of the Atlas

59

(C-1), the reader will only feel the transverses of the Atlas on each side just below and under the mastoid bone behind the ear. A misaligned Atlas will have one transverse distinctly tender on the side that it has misaligned toward. There are technically twelve possible misalignments of the Atlas, but for the reader's simplification, it should be determined as out to the left or right side. The adoption of a general correcting technique will be given for the Atlas in a later chapter.

Part Two of this chapter is concerned with feeling the spine in motion. Techniques for motion feeling of each area of the spine are as follows:

1. Motion Feeling of Pelvis (sacraliliac articulations)

Stand behind the person to be checked, looking at the back of his or her head and keeping a mental picture in your mind of what you are feeling. Place each thumb on each side of the sacraliliac articulations (dimples) and flare the rest of your fingers over each ilium. Ask the person to raise his or her right leg and pump with that leg somewhat like riding a bicycle. Then put the right leg down and do the same with the left leg all the time keeping your thumbs and fingers in place. Movement of these joints is not great, but if one side moves less than the other or not at all, that side is misaligned. The person will usually confirm this as he or she will feel some tenderness or pain on the involved side.

2. Motion Feeling of the Lumbar Vertebrae

Begin by finding L-4 lumbar spinous which can usually be detected at or near the same level as the sacraliliac articulations (dimples). With the person standing, move to his or her side and place your fingers on the L-4 spinous. Move down one spinous and your fingers will be on L-5 spinous. Ask the person to bend forward and then to each side as far as he or she can, keeping your fingers on the spinous of L-5. Do this with each of the five lumbar spinouses. As the person moves in each direction, you should be able to feel each spinous move. If any spinous has limited movement in comparison to other spinouses, or does not move at all, a misalignment of that vertebra is indicated.

3. Motion Feeling of the Thoracic Vertebrae

Side note: If you are right-handed, those fingers are already more sensitive, and visa versa if you are left-handed. This is the hand that should be used to do most of the feeling.

Now with your fingers on T-12, ask the person to slump and slouch completely forward, shoulders, head and all, and then slowly straighten to an erect position again. Do this with each spinous from T-12 up to T-1. Each spinous should move, and if any are limited relative to how the others move, then here again is a misalignment.

4. Motion Feeling of the Cervical Vertebrae

Have the person sit erect while standing at his or her side. Place one hand firmly on top of his head and the fingers of your other hand on C-7 spinous. The person should completely relax allowing you to support the head with your other hand. Move his or her head forward, chin to chest, and as you feel every spinous this way, each one should move *outward toward your fingers.* Next, move the head backward as far as possible, and your fingers should feel each spinous move *inward and away from your fingers.*

Next, keeping one hand on top of the head, find the lamina of C-2. With the thumb of your right hand on the left lamina, move the head from side to side checking the movement. Do this check for each of the cervical vertebrae, C-2 and below. Now stand to the right side of the person and change hands and repeat movements, feeling the lamina of each vertebra. To conclude motion feeling of the cervical vertebrae, gently rotate the head in each direction while standing at either side. All movements of the cervical spine should be smooth and equal in all directions, relative to what is a normal range of motion for that individual. The right and left transverses of the Atlas (C-1) can be felt under and just forward of the mastoid. Each transverse should move a little upon side to side as well as rotation movements of the head. Any limitations of the cervical spine should be noted. In fact, I suggest that a small notebook be purchased for each member of the family and that notes and comments be made regarding any tenderness or any motion feeling limitations associated with specific vertebrae.

At this point I would like to say that older people, sixty and older, who have never had their spines corrected regularly, will quite often have a more restricted range of motion in all areas of the spine. With this consideration kept in mind, expect less movement when feeling the spine of older members of the family but look for vertebrae that are moving less than the other vertebrae located in the same general area. These individuals will also require a much easier correction with less force applied.

In summary of this chapter I would like to focus on the facts of learning something new. It is most important that you study basic anatomy. With new knowledge gained through self-education, you will develop confidence and competence necessary to apply the techniques outlined herein. The key to developing confidence is repetition. For example, when the multiplication tables were presented to you for the first time in school, you had to repeat, practice and visualize them in your mind. Once you mastered the multiplication tables, they could never be taken from you. Work seriously in understanding and applying the contents of the *Home Chiropractic Handbook*. Endeavor to understand the life principle working through the human form and study diligently all phases in applying the art of chiropractic in finding and correcting spinal nerve interference. At some point you will be able to apply these techniques whenever necessary, just like the multiplication tables.

In concluding this chapter, I offer this exercise to develop your intuitive feeling when checking the spine. "Old time" chiropractors used to practice this exercise diligently. Take one human hair and place it on a smooth surface such as marble or glass or any other perfectly smooth surface. Then place one piece of paper over the hair and try to feel and find that one hair with your fingers. When you can feel and find that one hair under a ream of one hundred sheets of paper, you will have developed intuition with regard to physical sensitivity.

Chapter 5
Spinal Correcting Techniques Applied

If you have read the previous four chapters and studied chapters Three and Four thoroughly, and understand them, you are now ready to learn to correct ("to make or set right") spinal misalignments. However, it should be clear, that the author of this handbook is not responsible for any injury or any health problems resulting from incorrectly copying or applying the techniques described and shown herein. This handbook was conceived and written with sincerity. Everything explained will benefit all who can accept responsibility for their own health.

The following two points must be considered before a spinal correction is made:

I. **When to correct:** If you have located a tender area on a family member's spine or if there appears to be a limitation of normal motion relative to the rest of the person's spine this is an indication a correction is needed.

II. **When not to correct:** If the family member complains of extreme pain and if the person suffered an extreme traumatic injury, see a professional.

A precise understanding of the next four factors is of paramount importance in giving an effective spinal correction. Each will be discussed and defined separately and then combined into one idea for memorization.

1. *Direction or Line of Drive.* As you will copy these techniques by observing the following photographs, the right direction or line of drive must be determined first. I will describe the proper direction for each correcting technique. However, each person is a uniquely shaped individual and the line of drive will vary with each person.

2. *Pressure.* After you are set up with the right direction or line of drive, apply pressure with your contact hand or hands bringing the general area to tension, while maintaining the predetermined line of drive. This is very important.

3. *Force.* The amount of force needed must be determined by common sense. If the individual is relatively large with a muscular build, it may take considerable force; however, if the individual is small in stature, less force will be needed. With older people and children, very little force is needed. In fact, it is advised that you utilize just a little force with all corrections. When you develop confidence, you will know if and when to increase the amount of force. Force is relative to muscle tonus and size.

4. *Speed.* Speed is a compliment to force. As a general rule, the more speed you develop in correcting vertebrae, the less force you will need. Speed is relative to nothing, hence, the faster the better. Speed is especially appreciated by persons with much tenderness or pain. Note carefully, *force with speed should only be initiated after the area has been brought to tension. In this way you are not jolting the person when you follow through with the correction.*

These four major factors are aspects of one comprehensive concept. Visualize the following idea in its totality before making any correction. *It takes the right direction, applying pressure to a point of tension, providing sufficient force with speed, to set the vertebra in motion and reestablish its normal position.*

The following photographs will indicate the line of drive for each technique. All you need to do is copy the exact positions. When you follow through and make the correction, you should always feel and often hear the vertebra move ("pop") into place. If you are not feeling and hearing a solid correction, vary your line of drive to a slight degree. Further, evaluate the other three factors.

It may take more speed or a little more force. However, if the vertebra does not move after you have varied the line of drive slightly in all directions, leave the vertebra alone. In the case of a vertebra that has been misaligned for a long time, it often takes repeated attempts over a period of several days or weeks before the vertebra will move into place. With a misalignment of this nature use very gentle force, repeating the correcting technique once a day and eventually you will feel the vertebra move into place. Remember to keep a notebook on each family member until you become thoroughly acquainted with each one's spine.

Due to medical programming, people often wonder if vertebrae that are "popped" will wear out from popping. This is a fallacy. Vertebrae and discs will only wear if there is a misalignment causing uneven pressure. Vertebrae that are routinely corrected are prevented from wearing out because they maintain proper alignment. An analogy could be made to a piece of machinery. If the gears of a machine are kept in proper alignment, the machine has a much longer life expectancy. It is the same with the spinal column. It is much more desirable to have vertebrae (as well as all other joints of the body) move easily rather than to be stiff and immobilized with misalignments.

As I have not shown the correcting of an infant's spine, I will take this opportunity to discuss the procedure. All babies should have their spines checked regularly with the rest of the family. Babies born breech or in other difficult deliveries, especially where forceps were used, need to have their cervical spines checked as soon as possible after delivery. A vertebral misalignment caused by the birthing process can severely alter the health of the baby, sometimes causing ill health to continue throughout life. Following are specific instructions for successfully correcting a baby's spine. However, you should seek professional chiropractic assistance with these procedures.

Correcting the atlas (C-1) vertebra in the baby's spine will usually cause the rest of the vertebrae in the cervical, thoracic, and lumbar regions to maintain normal alignment. Have baby lying on his back, face up. Stand at baby's head and cradle baby's head with your hands. Using your first finger of each hand, feel the tiny transverses of the atlas. If one transverse is over to one side more than the other and especially if baby cries with just very gentle pressure, then with a quick, very gentle force correct the atlas with the same finger. You may need to gently try different lines of drive. The vertebra will move easily and with very little force once you have discovered the correct line of drive.

Correct the thoracic and lumbar vertebrae by holding baby with one hand under the buttocks and having the front of baby's body against your chest, gently feel with the first and middle finger of your other hand, baby's full thoracic and lumbar spine. You will be able to feel if one spinous is off to either side. If a tender vertebra is located, the baby will usually cry or begin to squirm. With one finger on each side of the tender spinous, apply gentle and equal pressure, and with a quick, very gentle force the vertebra will "pop" into place easily. The thoracic and lumbar vertebrae can also be corrected with baby on his tummy. Using the tips of your thumbs, place them alongside each tender spinous and give a quick, very gentle force and the vertebra will "pop" into place easily.

The above baby correcting techniques may require that you change the line-of-drive slightly using very little force until the vertebra "pops" into place easily. With practice, these techniques will be easy to apply.

At this point it should be mentioned that prenatal care for pregnant women should always include spinal correcting. The baby's development not only depends on good nourishment and blood supply, but also proper nerve supply from the mother's nerve system to the uterus. This is essential. It is interesting to note that in the fetus, the brain and spinal cord are always the first organs formed.

All of the following correcting techniques can be easily applied for spinal maintenance care during pregnancy except those techniques that require the woman to lie on her stomach during the second and third trimesters. You should see a professional chiropractor during this time. Although there are many factors involved in proper care of the unborn child, by maintaining normal spinal alignment during pregnancy, the mother is helping to assure an easier delivery of a healthy baby.

I have given over one hundred thousand chiropractic spinal adjustments with much success, using the exact techniques in the following pictures. As a general rule I usually correct the thoracic region first, then the lumbar and/or pelvic regions and the cervical last. I always allow each patient to rest for five or ten minutes after all corrections have been made, and I recommend that you follow this procedure in your home. This allows the vertebrae time to stabilize in their normal position.

The last several photographs included in this chapter show my wife applying correcting techniques on our son, Jimmy, and myself. My wife is not a professional chiropractor, yet she has, through my instruction, provided me with *excellent* spinal care for a number of years prior to the publication of this book.

I will describe each correcting technique using the following terminology and further I will maintain the same order of explanation for each description. Thoroughly acquaint yourself with these terms, as this will enable you to apply correcting techniques in a much more proficient and accurate manner.

1. *Technique*—will describe how it is used and for which misalignment.
2. *Contact*—will describe hand or finger contact and where to place on spine.
3. *Line-of-drive*—will describe the direction that the correction is to be made toward.
4. *P.F.S.*—These letters will stand for Pressure, Force, and Speed. Each will be described together as pertaining to the specific correction shown.
5. *Observe*—indicates that you are to note the angle or other special points in the photograph.
6. *Stabilize*—This word will be used in describing the stabilization hand which does not make the correction but rather helps bring to tension, supports, lifts or adds stability.
7. *Follow through*—will describe the correction made to the line of drive.

67

At this point, I will also give you letter abbreviations used to describe the direction vertebrae have misaligned in, and further, the direction of the line-of-drive required to correct misaligned vertebrae.

P to A — is Posterior to Anterior meaning back to front.

S or Superior — means toward the head.

I or Inferior — means toward the feet.

S to I — Superior to Inferior meaning head to feet.

I to S — Inferior to Superior meaning feet to head.

Lateral — meaning to the side: left to right or right to left.

Perpendicular — means an angle of 90 degrees

Have the person whose spine is being corrected relax on the correcting table. If the person is in pain or is unable to relax, suggest that he visualize his body as being like a wet noodle. Holding this idea in mind for a short time will help the person to relax. To relax the cervical spine, suggest the head as being like a sack of beans. This visualization will help the person to relax his neck.

Follow all directions carefully. Practice these techniques until you become proficient in all of them, and you will find correcting the spine will be easy to do.

The following techniques are, of course, not all the techniques that professional chiropractors use; however, they are some of the most easy and practical ones to apply at home.

Photograph 1

I am pointing to the thenar eminence (ball of my hand) contact point.

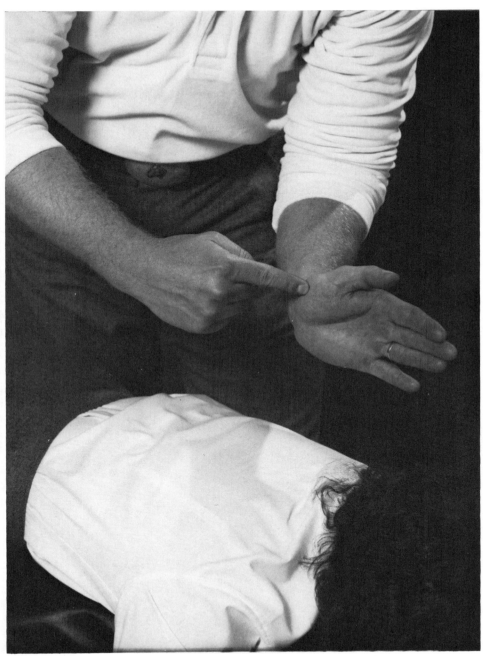

1.

Photograph 2

Technique—used to correct vertebra, T-1 through T-12, when misalignment is straight posterior.

Contact—thenar of each hand over right and left transverses of same vertebra.

Observe—equal positioning of my arms and hands. Depending on which thoracic vertebra you are correcting, reposition your stance alongside the person to maintain a similar line-of-drive relative to the shape of the person.

Line-of-Drive—P. to A., and a little superior.

P.F.S.—Apply pressure to tension, using a little force with speed, follow through maintaining line-of-drive.

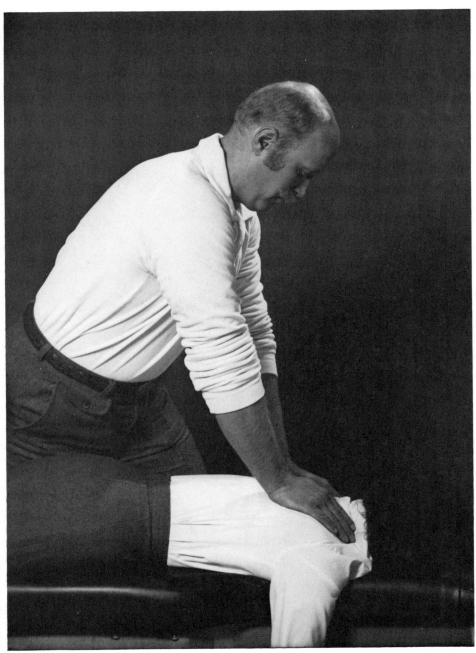

2.

73

Photograph 3

Technique — same as in Photograph 2.

Contact — same as Photograph 2.

Observe — Look down the middle of the person's body all the way to the heels. Note that the "V-shape" formed by my forearms is equal on each side of the person's body. This is important as it will accomplish an even line-of-drive for a precise P. to A. correction. Maintain this V-shape as you reposition yourself on any thoracic vertebra, T-1 through T-12.

Line-of-Drive — same as Photograph 2.

P.F.S. — same as Photograph 2.

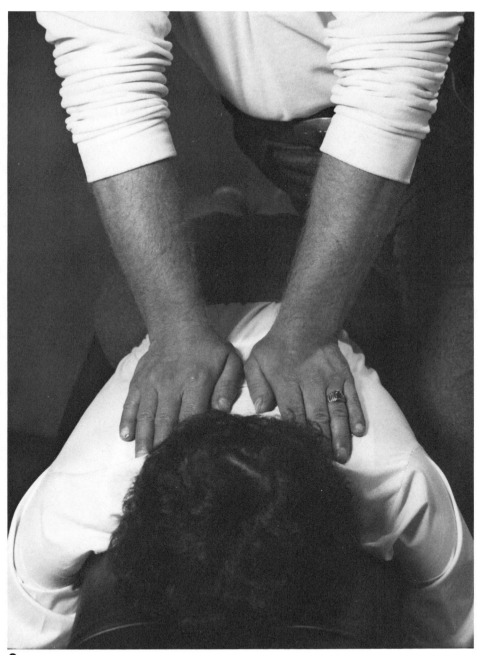

3.

Photograph 4

I am pointing to the pisiform bone (heel of my hand).

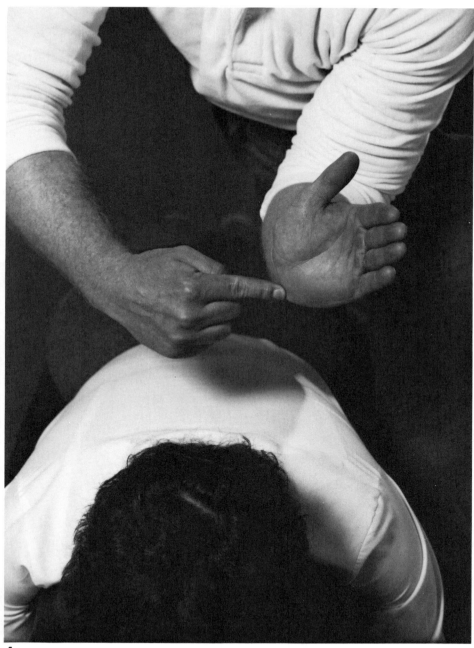

4.

Photograph 5

Technique — This technique is used to correct a vertebra, T-1 through L-5, that is misaligned having the whole vertebral body posterior with the right transverse low and the left transverse high.

Contact — pisiform of left hand on right transverse process; (note: ring is always on finger of my left hand). Pisiform of right hand on opposite transverse stabilizing with pressure.

Observe — my left hand and left forearm are exactly perpendicular (90 degrees to the person's body). Note my wrists are together and my hands form a 90 degree angle with each other.

Line-of-Drive — left hand drives P. to A. and Superior.

P.F.S. — Apply pressure to tension with both hands, right hand stabilizes, left hand uses a little force with speed following through line-of-drive.

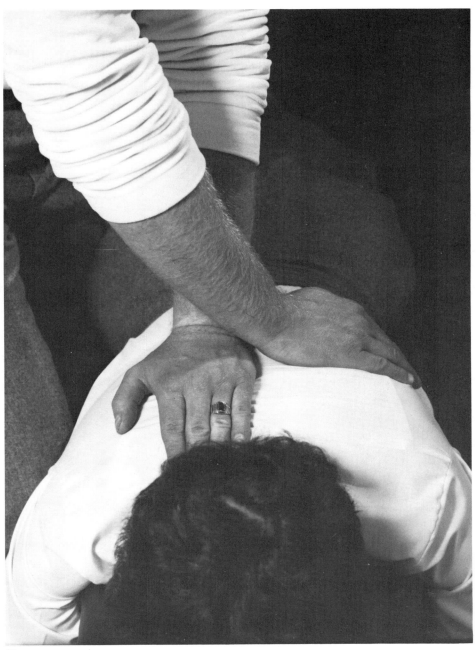

5.

Photograph 6

Technique — Lateral view of same technique in Photograph 5.

Contact — same as Photograph 5.

Observe — Right arm is perpendicular to person's body, right hand is stabilizing with pressure. Remember to reposition your stance alongside the person to maintain line-of-drive relative to the shape of the individual.

Line-of-Drive — same as Photograph 5.

P.F.S. — same as Photograph 5.

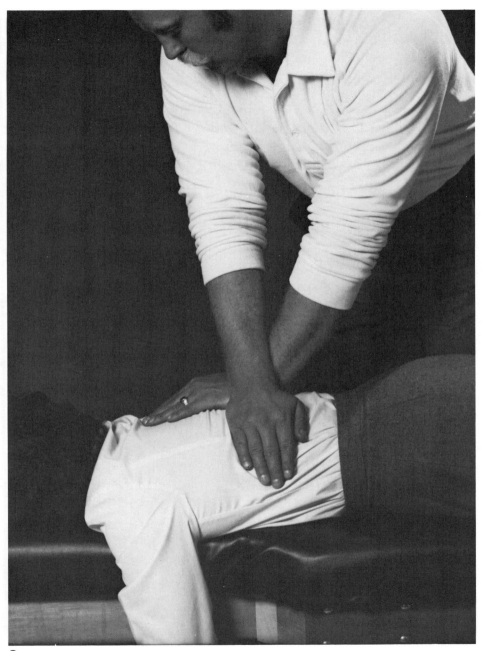

6.

Photograph 7

This photograph and Photograph 8 are showing the same technique as in Photographs 5 and 6. I have moved to the opposite side of the person's body reversing my contact hands.

Technique—This technique is used to correct a vertebra, T-1 through L-5, that is misaligned having the whole vertebral body posterior with the left transverse low and the right transverse high.

Contact—pisiform of right hand on left transverse process; pisiform of left hand on opposite transverse stabilizing with pressure.

Observe—my right hand and right forearm are exactly perpendicular. Note my wrists are together and my hands form a 90 degree angle with each other.

Line-of-Drive—right hand drives P. to A. and Superior.

P.F.S.—Apply pressure to tension with both hands, left hand stabilizes, right hand uses a little force with speed following through line-of-drive.

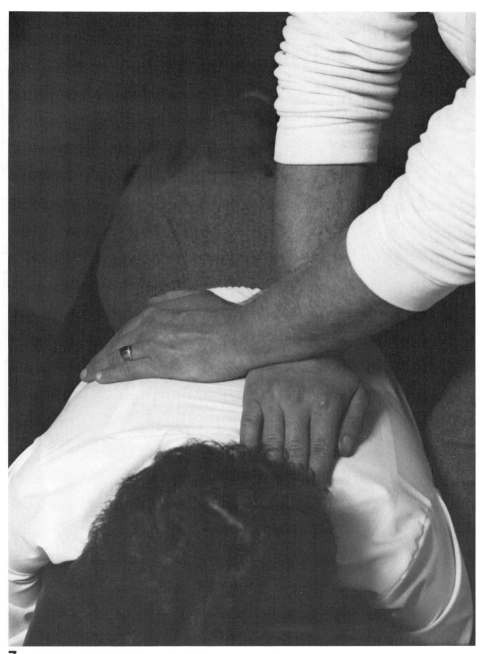

7.

Photograph 8

Technique—Lateral view of same technique in Photograph 7.

Contact—same as Photograph 7.

Observe—Left arm is perpendicular to person's body, left hand is stabilizing with pressure.

Line-of-Drive—same as Photograph 7.

P.F.S.—same as Photograph 7.

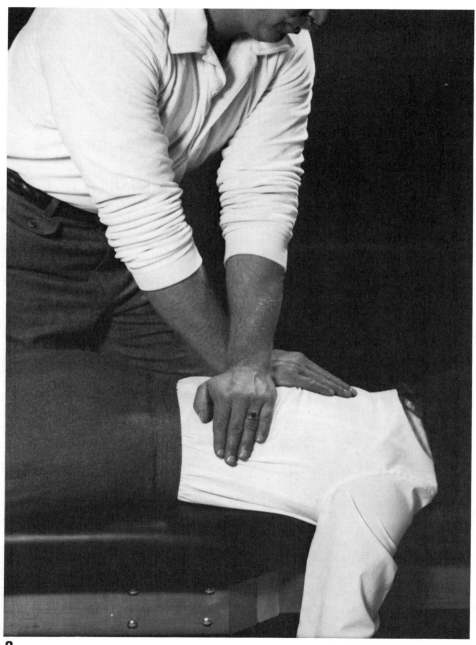

8.

Photograph 9

Technique—This technique is used to correct a vertebra, T-1 through L-5, that is misaligned having the vertebral body superior and posterior, with the left transverse high and the right transverse low.

Contact—pisiform of left hand on left transverse process; with pisiform of right hand on right transverse stabilizing with pressure.

Observe—Left contact hand is perpendicular to person's body.

Line-of-Drive—Left hand drives P. to A. and Inferior.

P.F.S.—Apply pressure to tension with both hands; right hand stabilizes, left hand uses a little force with speed, following through with line-of-drive.

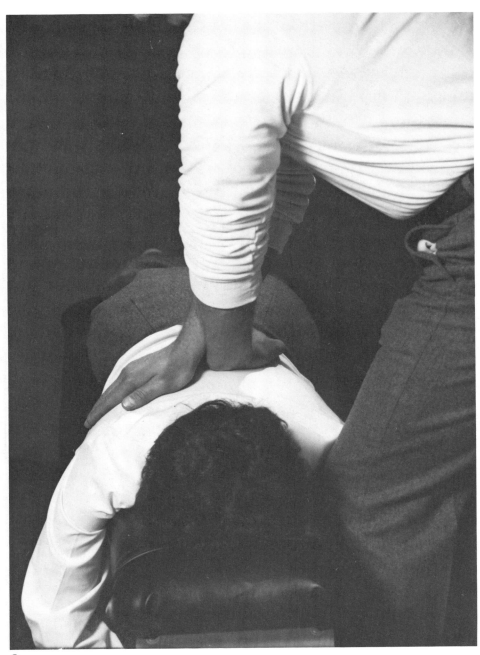

9.

Photograph 10

Technique — Lateral view of same technique in Photograph 9.

Contact — same as Photograph 9.

Observe — My wrists are together and my hands form a 90 degree angle with each other.

Line-of-Drive — same as Photograph 9.

P.F.S. — same as Photograph 9.

Technique Description for Right Side

Technique — This technique is also used to correct vertebrae, T-1 through L-5, that is misaligned having the vertebral body superior and posterior, with the right transverse high and the left transverse low.

Contact — Reposition yourself on the person's right side. Reverse your hands: pisiform of right hand on right transverse process; with left hand on left transverse stabilizing with pressure.

Line-of-Drive — Right hand drives P. to A. and Inferior.

P.F.S. — Apply pressure to tension with both hands; left hand stabilizes, right hand uses a little force with speed, following through with line-of-drive.

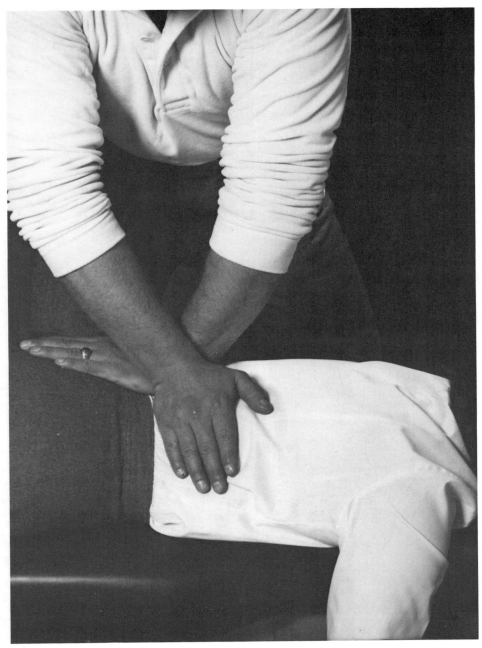

10.

Photograph 11

The following techniques with the person laying on his or her side for lumbar and pelvic correcting were once referred to as a "million dollar roll." This is because they provide great relief from lower back pain as well as restore normal nerve transmission. They are very simple and easy to copy.

Technique—Pull technique used in L-1 through L-5, for vertebra misaligned posterior with spinous to the right.

Observe—Have person lie on right side; left leg is bent forward with left foot tucked behind right knee; left foot must be kept firmly in place while correction is made.

Contact—middle finger of right hand firmly grasping lumbar spinous.

Line-of-Drive—I am pulling laterally (lifting spinous up toward me).

P.F.S.—Apply pressure to tension with knee of your right leg on top of person's left leg; at same time apply pressure to tension with your left hand stabilizing on the person's left shoulder. To make correction with your contact hand and finger, pull to tension using a little force with speed, following through line-of-drive.

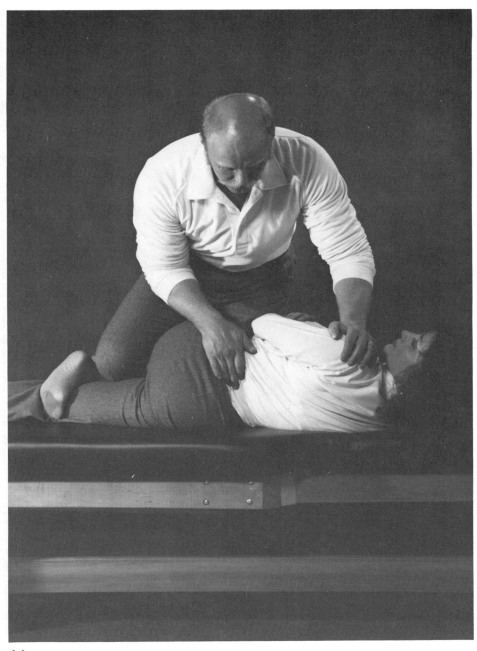

11.

Photograph 12

Technique — Pull technique used in L-1 through L-5, for vertebra misaligned posterior with spinous to the left.

Observe — Have the person lie on left side; right leg is bent forward with right foot tucked behind left knee; right foot must be kept firmly in place while correction is made.

Contact — middle finger of left hand firmly grasping lumbar spinous.

Line-of-Drive — I am pulling laterally (lifting spinous up toward me).

P.F.S. — Apply pressure to tension with knee of your left leg on top of person's right leg; at same time apply pressure to tension with your right hand stabilizing on the person's right shoulder. To make correction with your contact hand and finger, pull to tension using a little force with speed, following through line-of-drive.

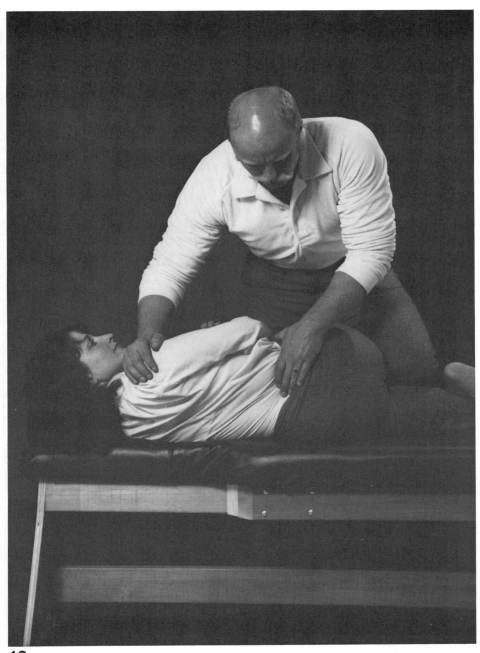

12.

Photograph 13

Technique — Pull technique used to correct posterior left ilium (ilium that has misaligned backward on sacrum).

Contact — middle 3 fingers of my right hand firmly grasping person's posterior crest of left ilium.

Observe — person is in same position as in Photograph 11.

Line-of-Line — I am pulling laterally (lifting ilium up toward me).

P.F.S. — Apply pressure to tension with knee of your right leg on top of person's left leg; at same time apply pressure to tension with your left hand stabilizing on the person's left shoulder. To make correction with 3 fingers of your contact hand, pull ilium to tension using little force with speed, following through line-of-drive.

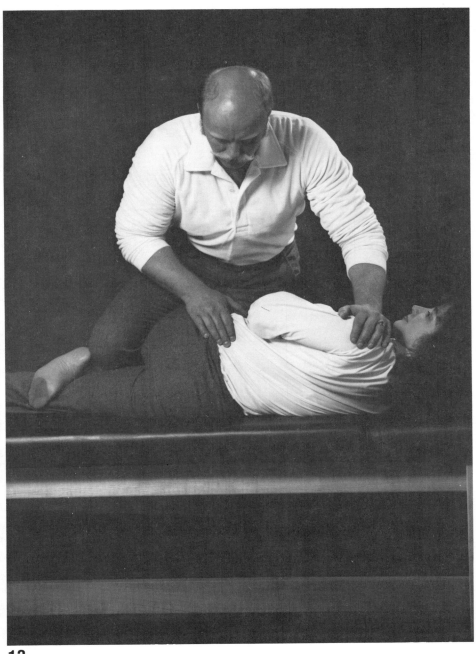

13.

Photograph 14

Technique — Pull technique used to correct posterior right ilium (ilium that has misaligned backward on sacrum).

Contact — middle 3 fingers of my left hand firmly grasping person's posterior crest of right ilium.

Observe — person is in same position as in Photograph 12.

Line-of-Drive — I am pulling laterally (lifting ilium up toward me).

P.F.S. — Apply pressure to tension with knee of your left leg on top of person's right leg; at same time apply pressure to tension with your right hand stabilizing on the person's right shoulder. To make correction with 3 fingers of your contact hand, pull ilium to tension using little force with speed, following through line-of-drive.

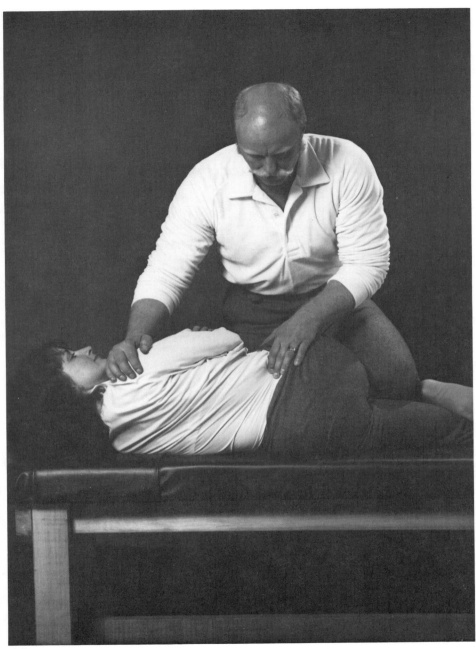

14.

Photograph 15

Depending on contour or shape of person, this push technique shown in Photographs 15 and 16, may be more effective than previous pull technique for same posterior left and right ilium misalignments.

Technique—Push technique used to correct posterior left ilium (ilium has misaligned backward on sacrum).

Contact—right hand pisiform contact on person's posterior crest of left ilium.

Observe—my right forearm is 90 degrees to person's body.

Line-of-Drive—push straight P. to A.

P.F.S.—Apply pressure to tension with knee of your right leg on top of person's left leg; at same time apply pressure to tension with your left hand stabilizing on the person's left shoulder. To make correction with your pisiform hand contact, push to tension using a little force with speed, following through line-of-drive.

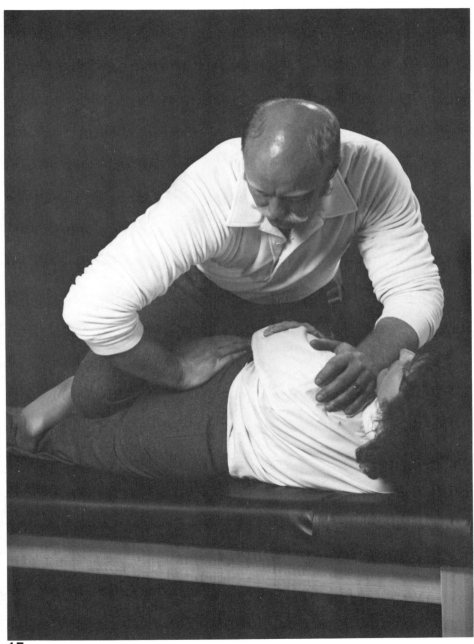

15.

Photograph 16

Technique — Push technique used to correct posterior right ilium (ilium has misaligned backward on sacrum).

Contact — left hand pisiform contact on person's posterior crest of right ilium.

Observe — my left forearm is 90 degrees to person's body.

Line-of-Drive — push straight P. to A.

P.F.S. — Apply pressure to tension with knee of your left leg on top of person's right leg; at same time apply pressure to tension with your right hand stabilizing on the person's right shoulder. To make correction with your pisiform hand contact, push to tension using a little force with speed, following through line-of-drive.

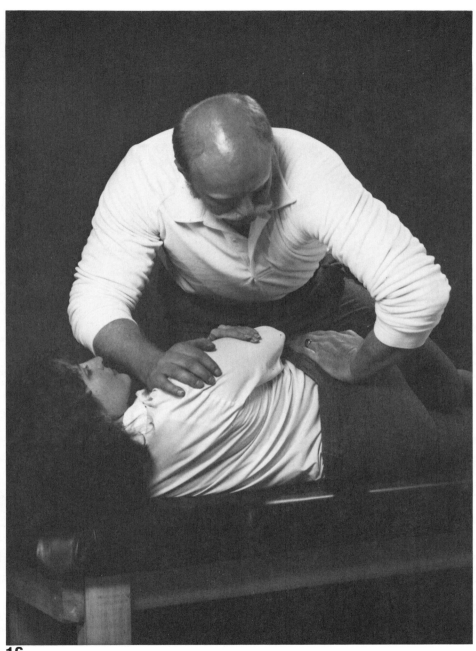

16.

Photograph 17
Leg Check—Part I

Photos 17 and 18 show parts I and II of the leg check that was described for you in Chapter Four (pages 58-59). Refer back to the description and note the position of my hands as I hold her ankles and check for equal length. Reread this leg check carefully as it will help in determining which of the proceeding techniques to apply.

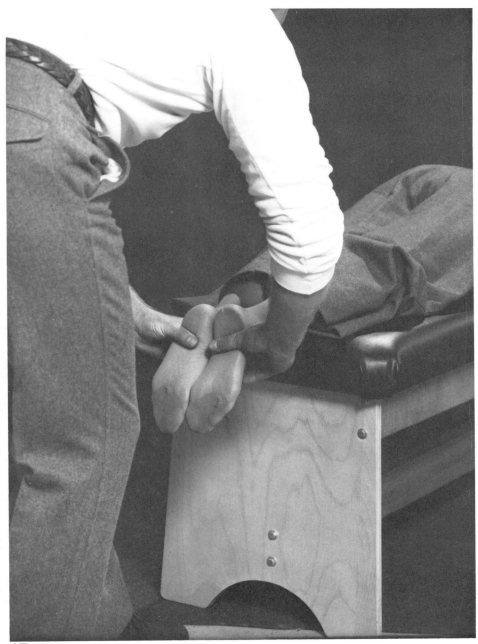

17.

Photograph 18
Leg Check — Part II

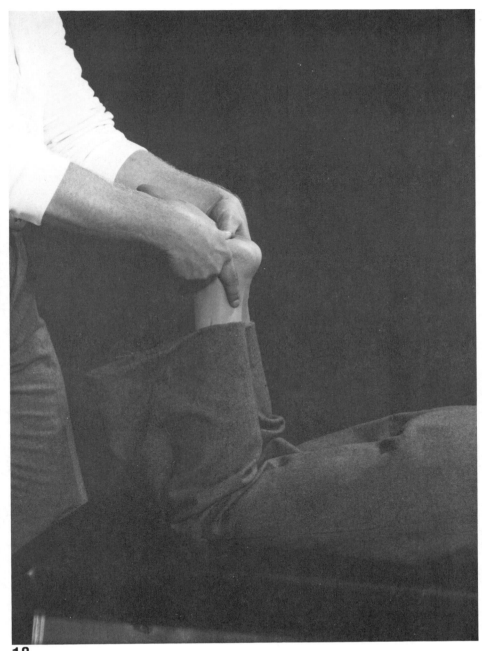

18.

Photograph 19

Technique — Push technique for double P.I. iliums (meaning both hips have misaligned to posterior and inferior positions).

Contact — Thenar of each hand on corresponding posterior crest of each ilium.

Observe — Equal positioning of my arms and hands.

Line-of-Drive — P. to A. and Superior.

P.F.S. — Bring pressure to tension using a little force with speed following through line-of-drive.

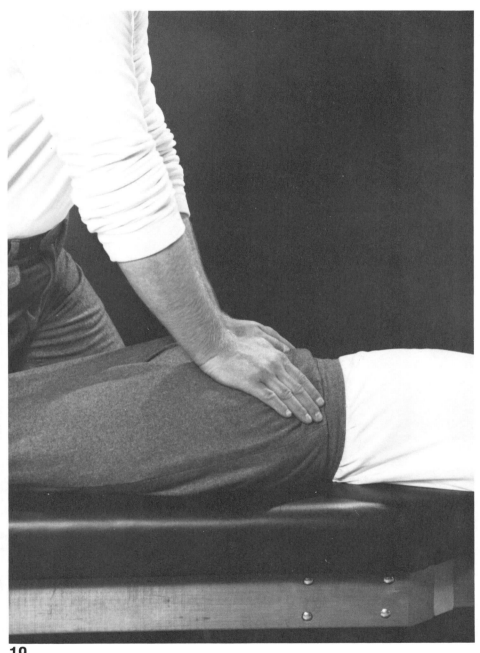

19.

Photograph 20

Technique—Push technique for A.S. left ilium (hip has misaligned to the front and high on the left side; leg is short on left side).

Contact—pisiform of left hand on top part of posterior crest of person's left ilium; pisiform of right hand on bottom part of posterior crest of right ilium.

Observe—the even angle formed by my upper and lower arms; my hands are exactly parallel to each other.

Line-of-Drive—Left hand drives inferior and a little P. to A. Right hand drives superior and a little P. to A.

P.F.S.—Apply pressure equally in opposite directions to tension, using a little force with speed drive contact points in opposite directions, following through line-of-drive.

Technique for A.S. Right Ilium

Technique—Push technique for A.S. Right Ilium (hip has misaligned to the front and high on the right side; leg is short on right side).

Contact—Stand on same side of person; reverse hands on opposite iliums; pisiform of left hand on top part of posterior crest of person's right ilium; pisiform of right hand on bottom part of posterior crest of left ilium.

Observe—same as in Photograph 20.

Line-of-Drive—same as in Photograph 20.

P.F.S.—same as in Photograph 20.

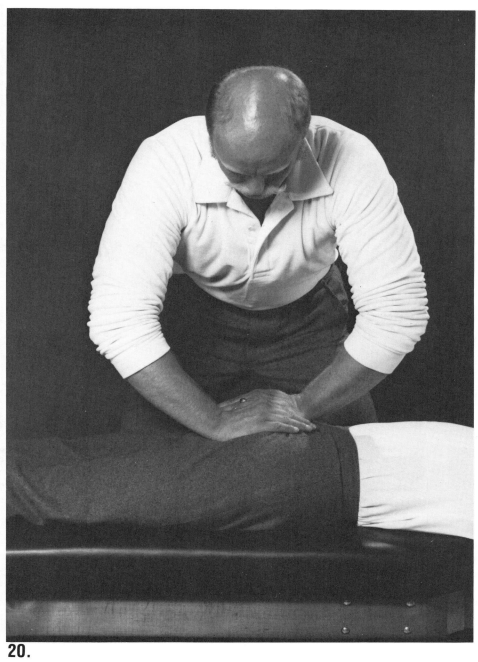

20.

Photograph 21

Technique — another push technique for A.S. left ilium (hip has misaligned to the front and high on the left side; leg is short on left side; also person will tend to have a "pigeon-toed" left foot, pointed inward).

Contact — pisiform of right hand on posterior crest of left ilium.

Observe — left hand grasping left ankle; you may lift leg slightly for extra leverage.

Line-of-Drive — right hand drives inferior and a little P. to A.

P.F.S. — Apply pressure to tension with right contact hand; at same time, using left hand lift person's leg up slightly; using a little force with speed following through line-of-drive.

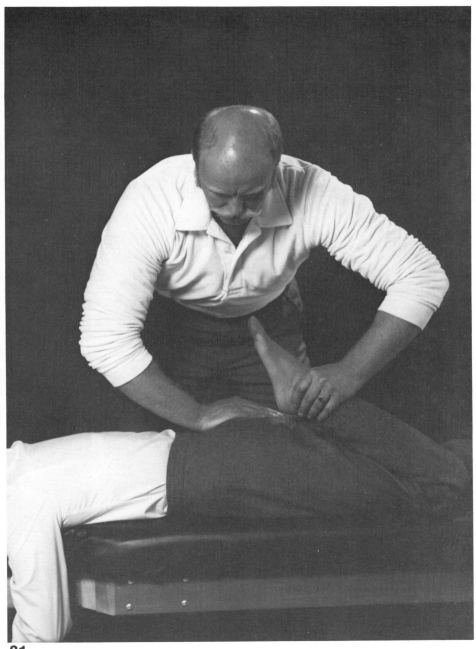

21.

111

Photograph 22

Technique — another push technique for A.S. right ilium (hip has misaligned to the front and high on the right side; leg is short on right side; also person will tend to have a "pigeon-toed" right foot, pointed inward).

Contact — pisiform of left hand on posterior crest of right ilium.

Observe — right hand grasping right ankle; you may lift leg slightly for extra leverage.

Line-of-Drive — left hand drives inferior and a little P. to A.

P.F.S. — Apply pressure to tension with left contact hand; at same time, using right hand, lift person's leg up slightly, using a little force with speed following through line-of-drive.

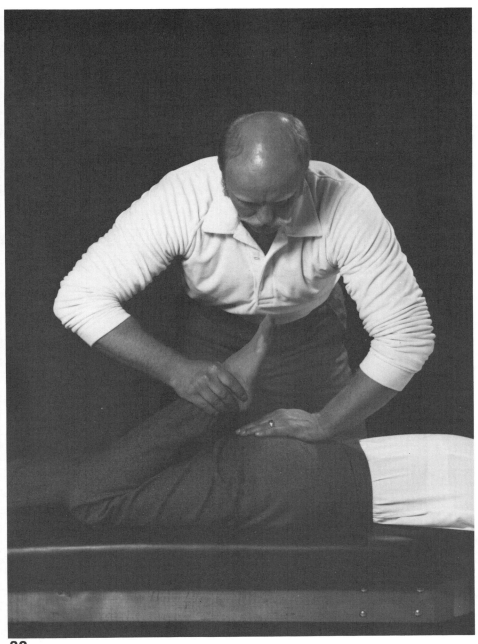

22.

Photograph 23

Technique—Push technique used for external left ilium (hip has rotated outward, causing left foot and toes to be pointed out to the side when standing).

Contact—pisiform of right hand on posterior crest of left ilium.

Observe—left hand grasping left ankle; you may lift leg slightly for extra leverage.

Line-of-Drive—right hand drives laterally away from you.

P.F.S.—Apply pressure to tension with right contact hand; at same time, using left hand, lift person's leg up slightly, using a little force with speed following through line-of-drive.

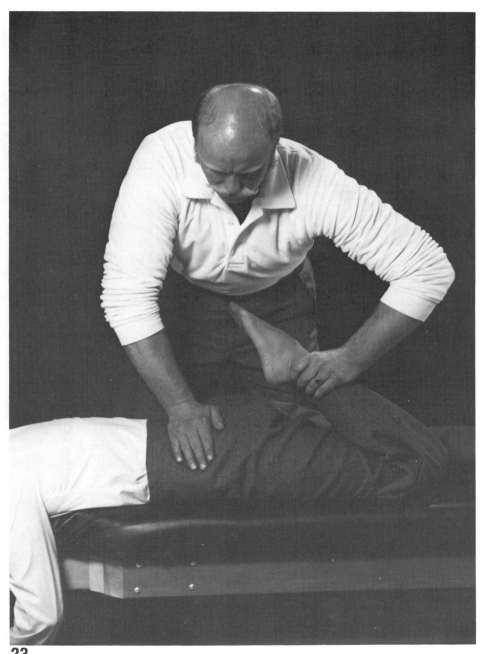

23.

Photograph 24

Technique — Push technique used for external right ilium (hip has rotated outward causing right foot and toes to be pointed out to the side when standing).

Contact — pisiform of left hand on posterior crest of right ilium.

Observe — right hand grasping right ankle; you may lift leg slightly for extra leverage.

Line-of-Drive — left hand drives laterally away from you.

P.F.S. — Apply pressure to tension with left contact hand; at same time, using right hand, lift person's leg up slightly, using a little force with speed following through line-of-drive.

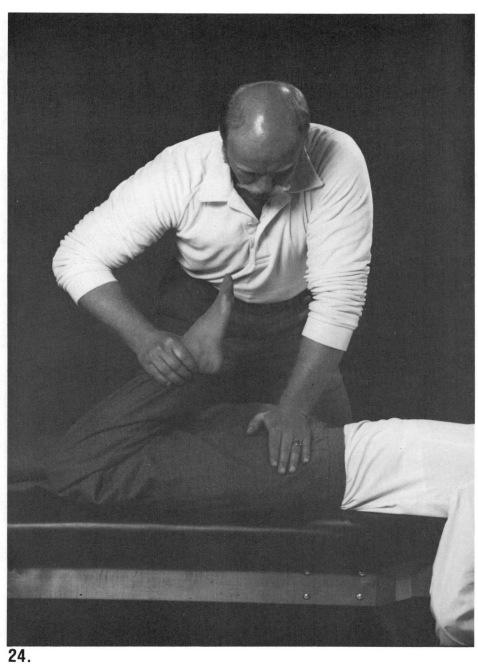

24.

117

Photograph 25

Technique—Push technique used for P.I. left ilium (hip has misaligned back and low on the left side.

Contact—pisiform of right hand on ishium of left hip.

Observe—right contact hand and forearm are exactly parallel to the person's body and correcting table for a direct superior line-of-drive.

Line-of-Drive—directly superior.

P.F.S.—Apply pressure to tension with knee of your right leg on top of person's left leg; at same time apply pressure to tension with your left hand stabilizing on the person's left shoulder; to make correction with pisiform on contact hand, bring to tension and using a little force with speed, following through line-of-drive.

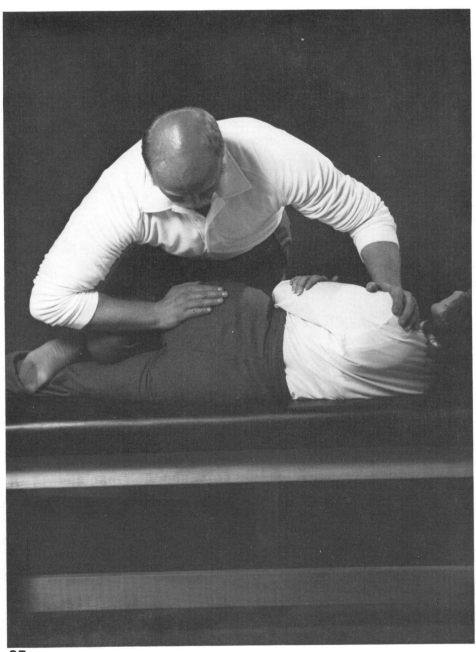

25.

Photograph 26

Technique—Push technique used for P.I. right ilium (hip has mis-aligned back and low on the right side.

Contact—pisiform of left hand on ishium of right hip.

Observe—left contact hand and forearm are exactly parallel to the person's body and correcting table for a direct superior line-of-drive.

Line-of-Drive—directly superior.

P.F.S.—Apply pressure to tension with knee of your left leg on top of person's right leg; at same time apply pressure to tension with your right hand stabilizing on the person's right shoulder; to make correction with pisiform on contact hand, bring to tension and using a little force with speed, following through line-of-drive.

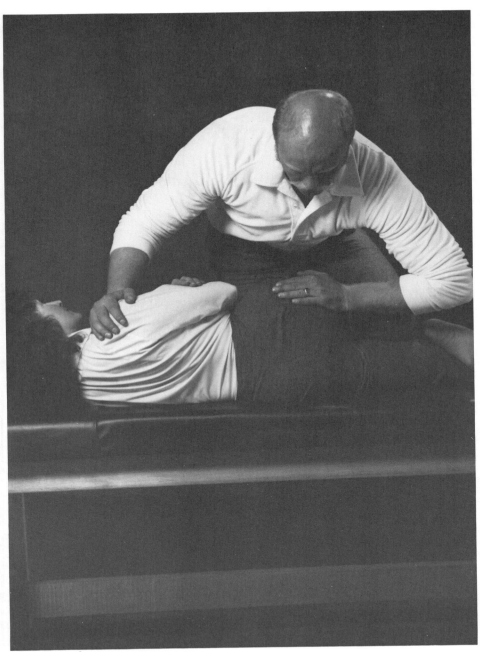

26.

Photograph 27

Technique — used for correcting posterior sacrum (sacrum has mis-aligned between iliums to the posterior).

Contact — Place your left hand on top of sacrum exactly between crests of iliums.

Observe — my right arm is perpendicular to the person's body.

Line-of-Drive — P. to A. and inferior.

P.F.S. — bring area to tension, using a little force with speed, following through line-of-drive.

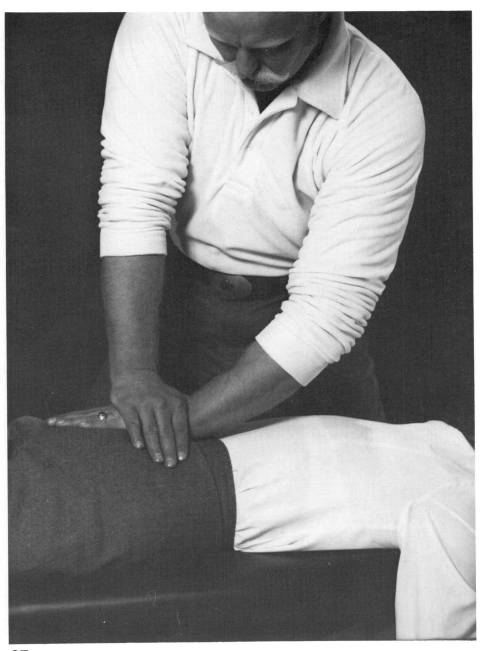

27.

Photograph 28

I am pointing to the first joint of my first finger (finger contact point 1).

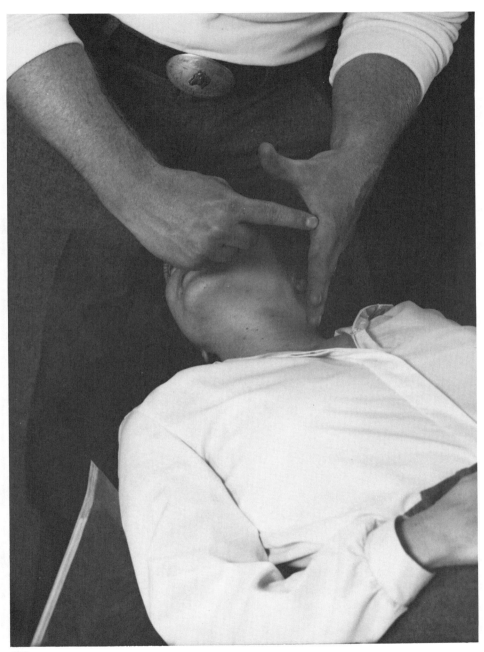

28.

Photograph 29

I am pointing to the second joint of my first finger (finger contact point 2).

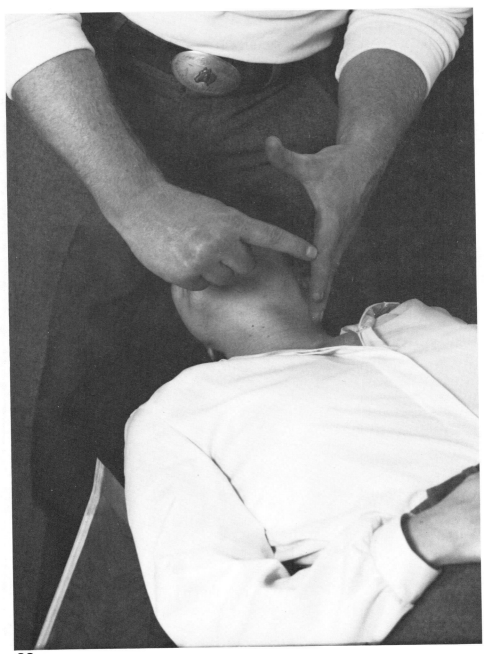

29.

Photograph 30

Technique—used to correct cervical vertebra: C-2, C-3, C-4. (vertebra misaligned with the vertebral body rotated to left and the spinous over to the right.

Contact—left hand using either finger contact: point 1 or point 2, on the lamina of C-2 or C-3 or C-4.

Observe—face turned to right side with right hand cradling head; left hand and forearm in straight line-of-drive across person's chest.

Line-of-Drive—laterally left to right and S. to I. at approximately 45 degree angle.

P.F.S.—**Important,** for all cervical correcting have the person completely relax. Suggest that he visualize his head is like a sack of beans, loose and floppy.

Lift head off the table, cradling the head with your right stabilizing hand, having the face turned to the right side, with your left hand finger contact on lamina, bring to tension using a little force with speed, following through line-of-drive.

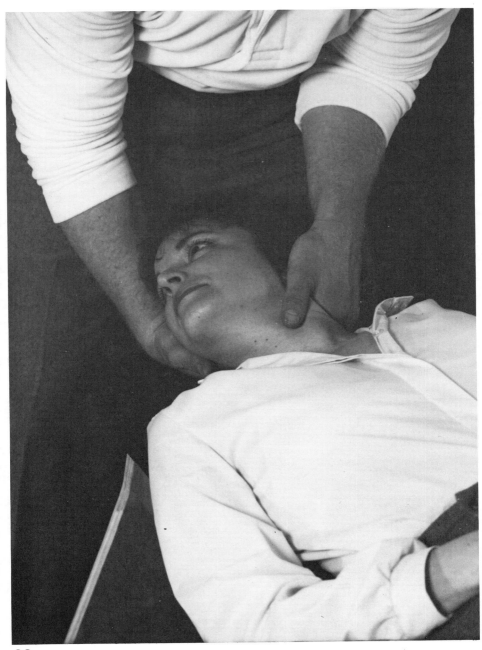

30.

129

Photograph 31

Technique — used to correct cervical vertebra: C-5, C-6, C-7. (vertebra misaligned with the vertebral body rotated to left and the spinous over to the right).

Contact — left hand using either finger contact: point 1 or point 2, on the lamina of C-5, C-6, C-7.

Observe — face turned to right side with right hand cradling head; left hand and forearm in straight line-of-drive across person's chest. For easy correction of lower cervicals C-5, C-6, C-7, the person's head is cocked up and more to the right side than in Photograph 30.

Line-of-Drive — same as in Photograph 30.

P.F.S. — same as in Photograph 30.

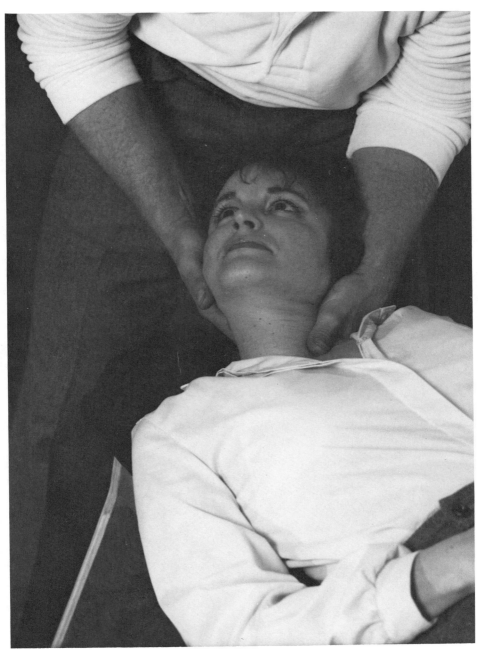

31.

Photograph 32

Technique — same technique as in Photos 30 and 31, but opposite side (vertebra misaligned with the vertebral body rotated to right and the spinous over to the left).

Contact — In this photo, finger point 1 is on C-4 lamina.

Observe — my right hand and forearm is in straight line-of-drive, 45 degrees across person's chest.

Line-of-Drive — laterally right to left and S. to I. at approximately 45 degree angle.

P.F.S. — Lift head off the table, cradling the head with your left stabilizing hand, having the face turned to the left side, with your right hand finger contact on lamina, bring to tension using a little force with speed, following through line-of-drive.

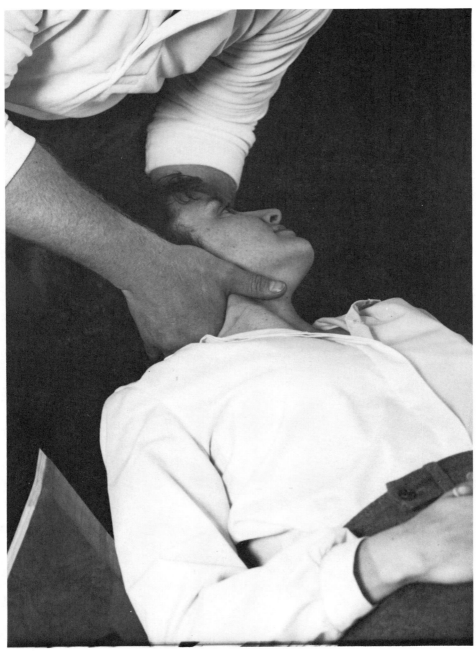

32.

133

Photograph 33

Technique — used for correcting Atlas (C-1); Atlas has misaligned laterally (out to left side).

Contact — left hand finger point 1 on left transverse of Atlas.

Observe — 90 degree angle formed by my contact hand and forearm with person's face and head.

Line-of-Drive — lateral, left to right and slightly S. to I., with angle of your arm no more than 90 degrees to the person's head (do not drive I. to S.).

P.F.S. — have person hold teeth together gently; stabilize jaw with your right hand and cradle head on forearm off table, having face turned to right side with left hand finger point contact 1 on left transverse of Atlas; bring to tension, using a little force with speed, following through line-of-drive.

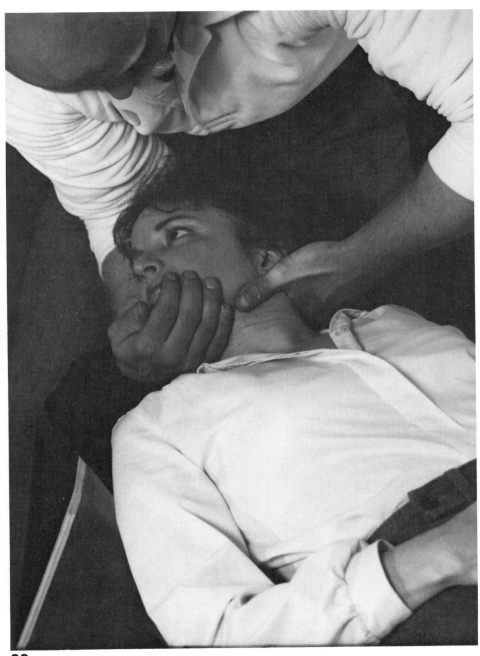

33.

Photograph 34

Technique—used for correcting Atlas (C-1); Atlas has misaligned laterally (out to right side).

Contact—right hand finger point 1 on right transverse of Atlas.

Line-of-Drive—lateral, right to left and slightly S. to I., with angle of your arm no more than 90 degrees to the person's head (do not drive I. to S.).

P.F.S.—have person hold teeth together gently; stabilize jaw with your left hand and cradle head on forearm, off table, having face turned to left side with right hand finger point contact 1 on right transverse of Atlas; bring to tension, using a little force with speed, following through line-of-drive.

I prefer the cervical techniques I have given you thus far; however, I shall include some more that I use occasionally.

136

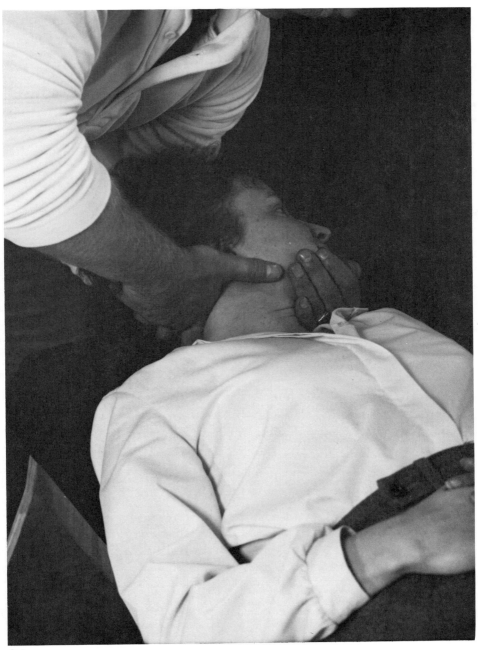

34.

Photograph 35

Technique— used to correct cervical vertebra, C-2 through C-7 (vertebra misaligned having vertebral body to right with spinous to left).

Contact— right hand finger point contact 2 on person's right lamina.

Observe— contact hand is approximately 90 degrees to the person's body.

Line-of-Drive— laterally, right to left.

P.F.S. — have the person's head turned to the left side, stabilize with your left hand over the person's head and face; with your right hand finger contact point 2 on right lamina of vertebra C-2 or C-3 or C-4 or C-5 or C-6 or C-7, bring to tension, using a little force with speed, following through with line-of-drive.

Same Technique — Opposite Side

To correct vertebra C-2 through C-7 misaligned having vertebral body to left with spinous to right, reposition yourself on opposite side of person. Person's head is turned to right side. Reverse your contact and stabilizing hands. Apply same P.F.S. except line-of-drive is left to right.

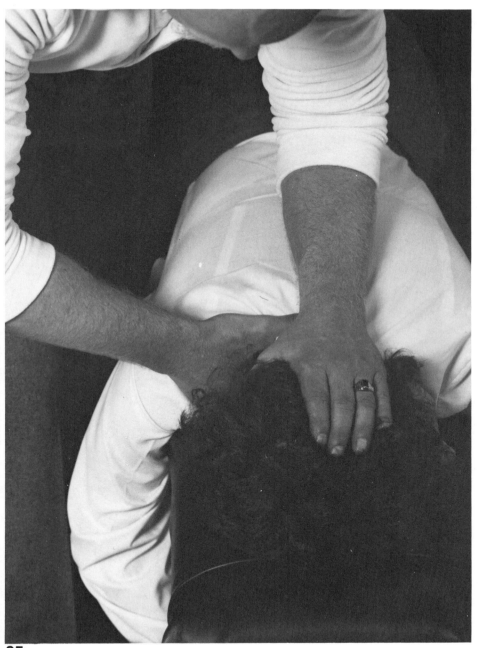

35.

Photograph 36

Technique — used to correct upper thoracic vertebra: T-1, T-2, or T-3 (that have misaligned with spinous to the right side).

Contact — pisiform of right hand on spinous.

Observe — contact hand is approximately 90 degrees to the person's body.

Line-of-Drive — laterally, right to left.

P.F.S. — have the person's head turned to the left side, stabilize with your left hand over the person's head and face; with your right hand pisiform contact on spinous of T-1 or T-2 or T-3, bring to tension, using force with speed, following through with line-of-drive.

Same Technique — Opposite Side

To correct upper thoracic vertebra: T-1, T-2, T-3 (that have misaligned with spinous to the left side), reposition yourself on opposite side of person. Person's head is turned to right side. Reverse your contact and stabilizing hands. Apply same P.F.S. except line-of-drive is left to right.

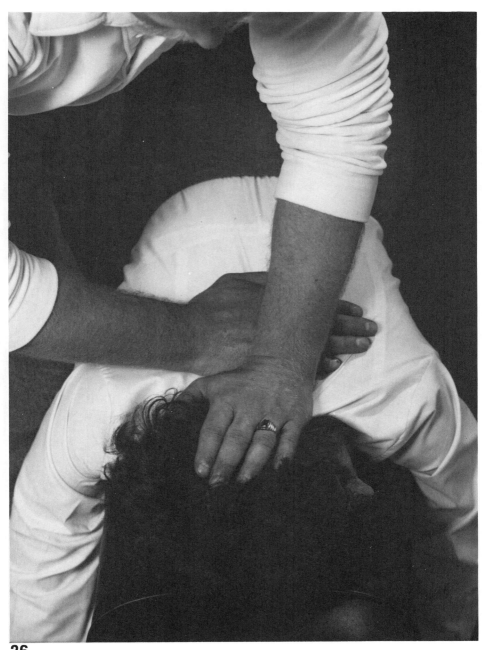

36.

Photograph 37

Technique—used to correct vertebra C-2 through C-7 (vertebra misaligned having vertebral body to right and spinous to left).

Contact—middle finger of left hand on lamina of any vertebra, C-2 through C-7.

Observe—left contact hand and forearm is parallel to the floor and 90 degrees to person's body.

Line-of-Drive—lateral pulling toward your body.

P.F.S.—stabilize with your right hand cradling person's right side of face and neck; with your left hand middle finger contact turn person's head to face you, bring to tension, using a little force with speed, following through line-of-drive.

Same Technique—Opposite Side

To correct vertebra, C-2 through C-7 (vertebra misaligned having vertebral body to left and spinous to right), reposition yourself on opposite side of person. Person's head is turned to right side. Reverse your contact and stabilizing hands. Apply same line-of-drive and same P.F.S. for opposite side.

142

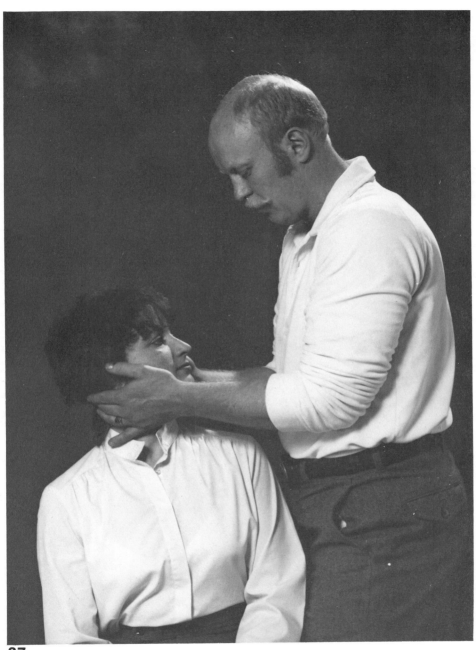

37.

Photograph 38

I am applying a spinal correcting technique to our son, Jimmy. The description of this technique is the same as Photograph 15.

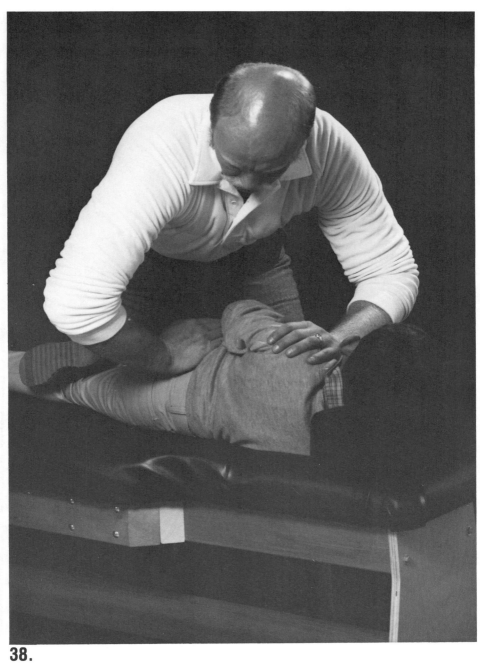

38.

145

Photograph 39

My wife is applying a spinal correcting technique to our son, Jimmy. The description of this technique is the same as Photograph 8.

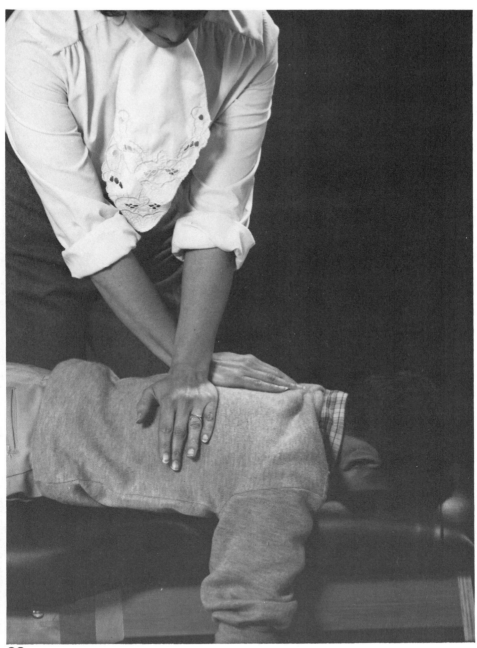

39.

Photograph 40

My wife is applying a spinal correcting technique to our son. The description of this technique is the same as Photograph 33.

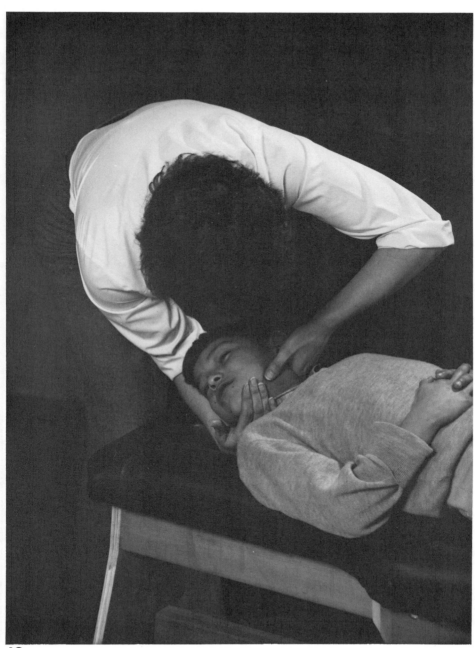

40.

Photograph 41

My wife is applying a spinal correcting technique to my cervical spine. The description of this technique is the same as Photograph 32.

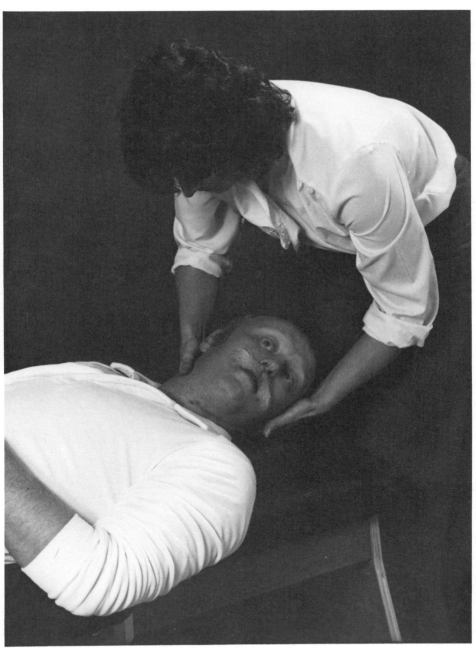

41.

Photograph 42

My wife is applying a spinal correcting technique to my lumbar spine. The description of this technique is the same as Photograph 11.

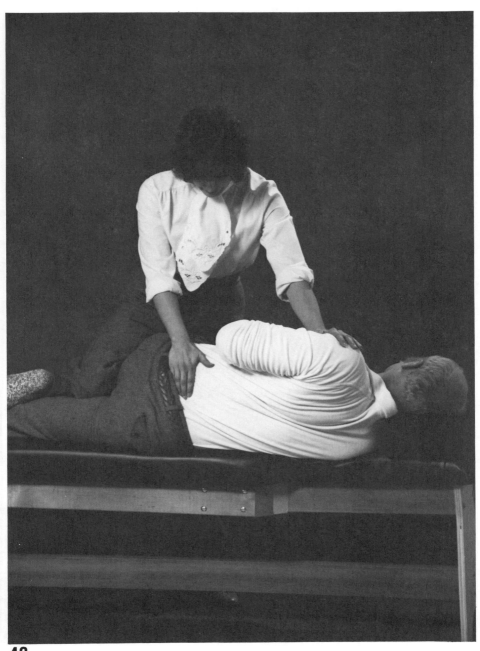

42.

Photograph 43

In conclusion of Chapter Five, the Holmquist family wishes you success in applying these correcting techniques in your own home.

If you and your family desire a more personalized approach, the Home Chiropractic Video is available. It brings the book alive and can make the application of the techniques so much easier for you.

Folks, I've put my heart into the making of this video. It is a full 100 minute professional production following the format of the book. It offers you the opportunity to actually see each technique demonstrated from different camera views. In addition, self-adjusting techniques are presented.

Because the most effective learning is accomplished through visual presentation, the Home Chiropractic Video will be an ideal learning tool for your entire family. It can greatly enhance your understanding and minimize the time required to learn the techniques and principle. I encourage you to order one today.

Available in any worldwide VHS format
For more information call 206-374-6500

Home Chiropractic Video - $49.^{95}
Washington residents add appropriate sales tax, please.

To order, clip form and send check or money order

- -

Amount enclosed $_____
Mail to:
Dr. Holmquist, One 8, Inc.
P.O. Box 2075 Dept. HCH
Forks, WA 98331-0822

Please send a Home Chiropractic Video to:

NAME_____

ADDRESS_____

_____

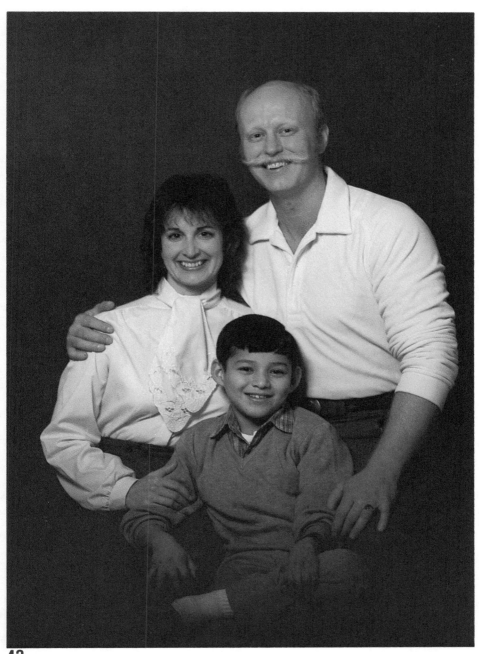

43.

Chapter 6
Build Your Own
Family Correcting Table

This chapter is intended to show you how to build a simple correcting table. The overall size of the table will be 5 feet long, 18 inches wide and 22 inches high. These dimensions were chosen to accommodate a family of average height and weight. The reason for the table being only 22 inches high is to provide leverage for making corrections.

A tall person should be able to lie face down with his or her knees supported on the table, while the feet hang over. This is important. If the feet do not hang over the table, they will turn to the sides and this tends to rotate the femurs (thigh bones) so that an accurate feeling of the pelvis is impaired. Children are so flexible that their feet can be supported by the table with toes pointing outward. However, it is recommended that a smaller version of the correcting table be constructed or purchased for spinal correcting of children.

Although the correcting techniques included in this book can be attempted on a firm bed or sofa, you can apply them with much greater competency, while using this simply designed table. It has the correct degree of firmness and allows the person whose spine is being corrected to assume a proper position.

Following is a list of tools and materials you will need to build your table. Tools required are as follows:

156

hammer   coping saw or jig saw
saw   paint brush
measuring tape   large screwdriver
square   razor blade
drill

Materials you will need:

1. 5 foot by 18 inch piece of ¾ inch thick plywood
2. Four 8-foot 2x4's
3. About 2 pounds of 16 penny galvinized nails or a box of 3 inch long screws (screws are stronger)
4. Sand paper
5. 8 feet by 3 feet piece of upholstery vinyl
6. 1 piece of 3-inch thick foam rubber, 5 feet 2 inches long by 20 inches wide
7. 1 box of large-head upholstery tacks or stapler
8. Paint or stain (color of your choice)
9. Contact cement

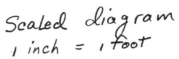

Scaled diagram
1 inch = 1 foot

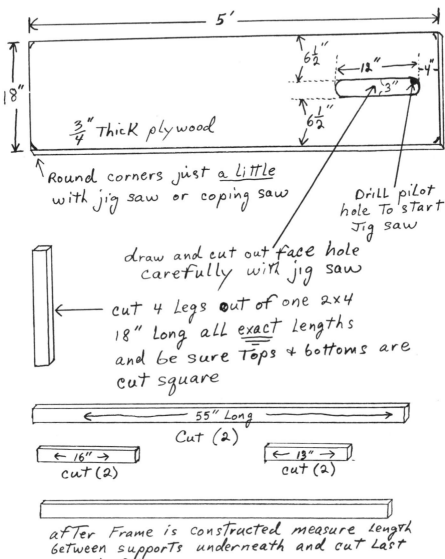

5'

18"

6½"

12"

4"

3"

¾" Thick plywood

6½"

Round corners just a little
with jig saw or coping saw

Drill pilot
hole To start
Jig saw

draw and cut out face hole
carefully with jig saw

cut 4 Legs out of one 2x4
18" Long all _exact_ Lengths
and be sure Tops & bottoms are
cut square

55" Long

Cut (2)

16"
cut (2)

13"
cut (2)

afTer Frame is constructed measure Length
between supports underneath and cut Last
2x4 to fit.

assembly diagram

Nail or screw top to frame,
a one inch Rim border will
extend over the frame all
the way around.

Sand corners and
sand frame

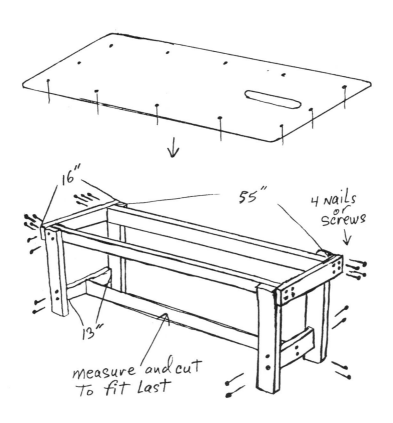

16"

55"

4 Nails
or
screws

13"

measure and cut
to fit last

Upholstery Instructions

1. Place foam rubber over the top of the table so it extends equally 1 inch all the way around the top.
2. Place a piece of upholstery vinyl 70 inches by 28 inches over foam rubber.
3. Begin by folding material under 1 inch (to eliminate raw edge) at foot of table. Tack or staple material beginning at center and working to each side. Next stretch, fold and tack material at head of table, in same manner.
4. Next, fold under material 1 inch and tack or staple from side to side keeping wrinkles out of material.
5. Cut a slit in the shape of an "H" over the face hole. The "H" slit should be 11 inches long and 3 inches wide directly over the face hole.
6. Fold under raw edge, pull and tack each flap of the "H" onto the bottom of the table, one flap toward the head and the other toward the foot of the table.
7. Cut 2 pieces of upholstery vinyl 15 inches wide by 18 inches long. Fold over and glue a 1 inch border along each 18-inch side to make a finished piece, 13 inches by 18 inches. Follow this procedure with both pieces.
8. Place 1 piece 13 inches by 18 inches, to right of face hole. Pull one end through face hole and tack to bottom of table. Pull tight and tack other end to bottom on outside rim of table. Follow this same procedure on left side of face hole with remaining piece, 13 inches by 18 inches.
9. Stain or paint the frame of the table a color of your choice.
10. Refer to Photograph Number One which shows this exact table.

To provide support for the neck and head when side-position corrections are given, use a pillow with the appropriate thickness for each individual's shoulders.

A step-up platform may also be required to enable a shorter individual to make spinal corrections. The frame for the step-up can be made from a 2" x 4" with a plywood top but with no legs attached. The step-up should be a reasonable size to stand on, approximately 4 feet long and 16 inches wide. A piece of carpet can be tacked to the top to provide secure footing. The platforms can be placed along side the correcting table and moved aside for a taller person. My aunt, Dr. Marion, used a step-up in her office.

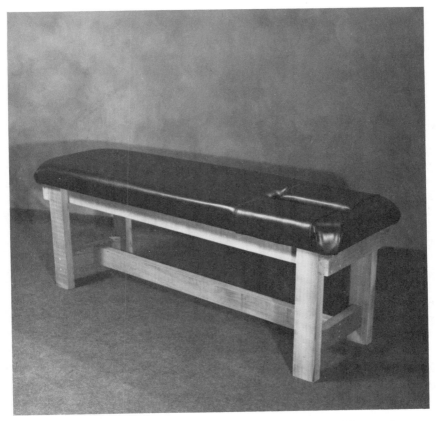

I strongly suggest that you either build the table as shown above or if you haven't acquired the necessary carpentry and upholstering skills, then you can order the table described on the following page. It is designed especially for use with this book and engineered to give optimum proficiency in correcting spinal mis-alignments.

Holmquist Chiropractic Table

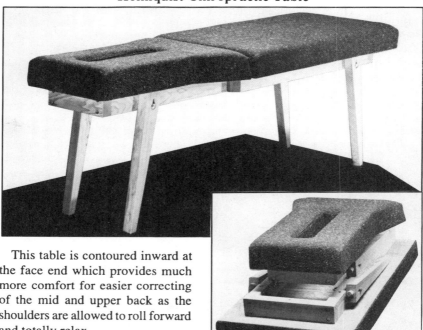

This table is contoured inward at the face end which provides much more comfort for easier correcting of the mid and upper back as the shoulders are allowed to roll forward and totally relax.

This fine table truly offers features that can make it much easier to locate and correct vertebral misalignments.

It's also great for giving a massage. Just sit alongside the person and transfer a nice relaxed feeling

To order, send check or money order to:

One 8, Inc.
Dept. HCH
P.O. Box 2075
Forks, WA 98331-0822

Current price is $495.00 and we pay shipping anywhere in the U.S. or Canada. Washington residents add appropriate sales tax.

Folds quick and easy to carry. It is shipped to you fully assembled. An attractive piece of furniture, it is finely crafted with a wooden frame and covered with a durable 100% nylon fabric that is washable. Color in stock is char-brown tweed which will compliment almost any decor.

For more information or any questions, just write or call:
1-206-374-6500

It's a worthwhile family investment!

Send personal check, wait 6 weeks.
Send money order, shipped to you within 5 working days.

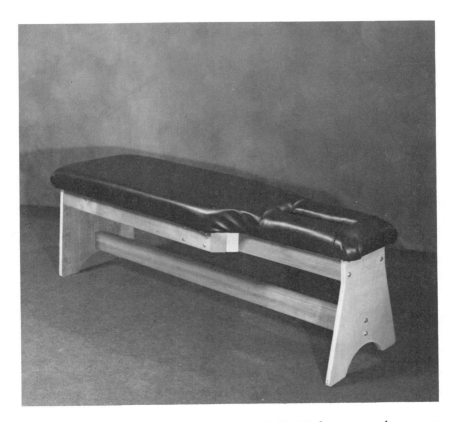

The Founder of Chiropractic, D.D. Palmer, used a very simply designed table and produced marvelous results. In fact, his first spinal adjustment in 1895 was made on a man named Harvey Lillard, who had a total loss of hearing. He was able to hear for the first time in seventeen years after he received an adjustment by D.D. Palmer. Furthermore, D.D. Palmer was a fish peddler who was self-taught in anatomy and physiology, and through self-discipline and study, discovered the life principle of chiropractic. Being a self-taught person is not like reading the evening paper. Rather, it is a diligent persevering study that becomes a priority in life. As in D.D. Palmer's example, other activities were set aside in order to perfect and apply the knowledge gleaned from his study. He was a very determined individual. He attracted patients and students by the hundreds and the profession of chiropractic grew rapidly.

Now, dear reader, it would seem that if one man can teach himself and use a simple table as D.D. Palmer did, then you also can be self-taught through a disciplined study of this handbook and use a simple table for application.

Chapter 7
Family Maintenance Correcting

Chiropractic care was originally developed with the idea of providing health maintenance in an intelligent manner. Before proceeding any further, the word "maintain" will be defined from *Webster's Dictionary*:

> 1: to keep in an existing state: preserve from failure or decline (--one's health) (--machinery) 2: to sustain against opposition or danger: uphold and defend (--a position) 3: to continue to persevere in: carry on: keep up.

It should be understood from previous chapters that chiropractic spinal correcting is a way to bring the entire body into a healthy state. If this is not understood, then reread over and over the previous chapters and thoroughly study the six major systems of the body, keeping in mind the brain and spinal cord is the master system that controls all other systems. Once the body is brought into a healthy state, then we should maintain that health by continual intelligent upkeep, which includes spinal correcting throughout one's life. Set aside a specific time each week for all family members to have their spines checked.

Children will usually respond very quickly to spinal correcting. This is due to the fact that a child's body is relatively "brand new." However, even adults, once having regained health, can maintain it through spinal correcting.

The medical approach to health care is not maintenance.

Rather, as it is generally practiced today, it should be classified as crisis therapy. Medical procedure begins with a diagnosis, which means to name a condition, disease or health problem and proceeds to treat that condition usually with drugs or surgery. The fact that the condition has been named (diagnosed) does not at all imply that the cause of the condition is known. This procedure treats the effect and in reality totally evades the question: What caused the body to malfunction and how can the cause of the malfunction be corrected?

People are led to believe when they take a drug such as aspirin, the drug is transmitted only to that part of the body intended to receive it. Television commercials for aspirin show a special tube from the stomach to the brain. This is misleading and absolutely not true! Every drug that is either swallowed by mouth or injected by needle is absorbed into the bloodstream and pumped to every organ, all tissue and ultimately to every cell of the body! Further, the drug may act upon some part or system of the body in a pernicious manner and as a result side effects are often experienced.

Regarding drugs, shots, and immunizations, the author of this handbook has had virtually none! According to conventional opinion, I should be dead. Due to regular chiropractic maintenance care since infancy, and knowledge of other health factors to be discussed in the last two chapters of this book, I am extremely healthy and robust in nature. This brings up the topic of immunization. If you were to plan a trip into the depths of an African jungle where malaria is common, you *may* consider receiving an immunization beforehand. As stated previously, I have never had any immunizations of any kind. The decision to have or not have immunizations is yours alone. I, of course, am not responsible for your decisions in regard to this issue. Consider this fact: If every cell in your body is functioning normally, how can you get sick? You would have a natural high resistance and natural high immunity! This is the primary objective of the chiropractic philosophy: to maintain a high resistance in the body. It should be known that your body makes every antibody, every drug and every chemical automatically in the exact quantity and perfect quality required for your unique individual needs. The inborn intelligence within the body does all this for you, providing you maintain your body in a healthy state.

I would like to bring to your attention the familiar idea of surgeons wearing masks and gloves during operations. If you were to obtain a surgeon's mask and hold it up to the light, you would be able to see light through it. As the mask covers the surgeon's nose and mouth, air must be able to pass through the mask or the surgeon would suffocate. Now, how big do you think germs (bacteria and viruses) are? They are hundreds of times smaller than a human hair! They are miscroscopic. Most likely one hundred bacteria could hold hands — so to speak — and fly through the surgeon's mask. I find this quite amusing considering the medical profession is aware of the microscopic size of these microorganisms.

The sterile surgical gloves so carefully wrapped in an air-tight plastic package become amassed with germs from the air as soon as the package is opened. They are now as contaminated as the surgeon's hands. If you were to take a cotton swab and wipe any item in a so called sterile room, you will find, upon examination under a microscope, thousands upon thousands of germs. Therefore, the foregoing foolishness could be eliminated. Note, however, it is recognized that proper sanitation is essential. All that is necessary is for the doctor to maintain cleanliness.

It should be noted that medical crisis therapy may be required if the body has not been maintained in health and if parts of the body have seriously deteriorated. However, drugs should be very carefully and discriminately prescribed by medical doctors only. Surgery to remove any organ should be considered only as a very last resort.

The medical profession is well equipped to play its role as the crisis therapy health profession, caring for all serious injuries and life-threatening emergencies. As soon as the body has healed sufficiently from any serious injuries, the spine should be checked and corrected as this will expedite the healing process to a more complete state.

To document my contentions regarding drugs, immunizations, and surgery, I suggest you read the book, *Confessions of a Medical Heretic* by Robert S. Mendelsohn, M.D. Dr. Mendelsohn has practiced medicine for over twenty-five years and has been the chairman of the Medical Licensing Committee for the State of Illinois, as well as holding many other prestigious positions. His book will fully elaborate on my contentions as to how drugs and surgery fit into the general health care system.

Through spinal maintenance correcting, one can maintain a high resistance in the body and live in harmony with the environment. It is impossible to kill all germs (such as bacteria and virus) in the world. There are enough germs in the room where you are reading this book, to kill off the entire human population in the state where you live. If the germ theory of disease were true, there would be no one alive to tell about it. Germs cannot cause disease in a healthy body where all cells are functioning normally. They can only attack a cell that has a low resistance from not functioning normally. Even cancer appears to only take hold in the cells of a body that are not functioning properly.

All cells of the body are replaced within a seven-year period except the brain and spinal cord. Consider heart and blood cells which live for only approximately ninety days. In a certain period of time you will have a whole new circulatory system, heart and all! The key to perpetual health, even during the aging process, is for new healthy cells to replace old worn out or sick cells. In this way disease will pass from the body. Consider further, there is not a single known disease that someone has not recovered from, indicating the life in the body heals the body. Thus it is substantiated that application of the chiropractic life principle is part of the key to maintaining health. A further elaboration on total health will be discussed in the last two chapters of this book.

In summary, set aside a time for checking and correcting the spine of each family member. Improvement in health may be gradual at first, but with continued study and practice in refining the correcting techniques, you may eventually achieve health. Each adult member of the family should read this handbook and then reread and explain as much of it as possible to their children. In conclusion, cooperative family participation in spinal maintenance correcting will most assuredly produce lasting benefits.

In the next chapter I will endeavor to portray the professional chiropractor in the highest light. However, this is difficult at the present time. While there are fine chiropractors who have the patients' welfare at heart, it is my opinion, the profession in general has placed professionalism and financial gain above principle, and in blind quest for "professional status," a great principle has been compromised.

Chiropractic is simple, my friends. So simple that the great early chiropractors built the foundation of the profession with very little formal education. They used simple tables and were inspired by envisioning a healthier world through chiropractic. I have heard it said that the early Palmer family never wanted a formal profession but rather that each chiropractor teach others how to correct the spine. Had this occurred, chiropractic would have become a universally accepted healing system. It would have become ingrained in the consciousness of people everywhere. The principle would have been preserved, and a higher understanding of health and life would have been promulgated throughout the world.

When a person has a new home built, he doesn't have to ask for a "medicine cabinet" in the bathroom. He gets one automatically. That is how deeply ingrained the idea of taking medicine is. It would be nice if someday a chiropractic table came with every home. It can only happen if the concept of home chiropractic is perpetuated.

Chapter 8
When to See A Professional Chiropractor and How to Choose One

It should be understood that this handbook will give to the reader the knowledge to become as proficient as one desires in applying the techniques outlined herein. However, you may determine from your study that professional chiropractic assistance is necessary. Moreover, if pain continues, or some internal organ continues to malfunction even after you have applied spinal correcting for a period of time, see a professional chiropractor.

The doctor of chiropractic is a professional trained to analyze and correct spinal misalignments. The six years of extensive education furnish the chiropractor with proficiency in detecting and correcting spinal misalignments: a field of expertise no other health care professional provides for the public.

The term "principled chiropractor" refers to the many conscientious chiropractors committed to educating their patients concerning the philosophy of chiropractic. A principled chiropractor is one who realizes his expertise in caring for the spine is unique. His sincere purpose is to explain the life principle operating through the nerve system.

The doctor of chiropractic will endeavor to analyze your spine with great competency. X-rays may be used to obtain a picture of the spinal column and can be worth a thousand words as they provide a blueprint for the chiropractor to keep in mind as the

170

adjustment is given. Generally, chiropractors are conservative with x-rays and usually do not x-ray all patients. With the exception of very traumatic accidents, children rarely need x-rays. Often the doctor of chiropractic will also utilize very sensitive heat detecting instruments to locate inflamed spinal nerve roots along the spinal column. His adjusting tables are very elaborate, capable of accommodating many severe spinal problems. The principled chiropractor, utilizing x-ray, spinal instruments, hand palpation, and adjusting tables is well equipped to provide your family with professional spinal health care.

Regarding nutrition, he will be more than willing to provide sound nutritional advice about the various types of foods. He may suggest exercise in a way that is suitable to you as an individual. And on your behalf, he will be willing to work interprofessionally in a reasonable manner.

The fees of the principled chiropractor will not be excessive, and if you ask him about a regular professional maintenance checkup for your entire family, he will offer a suitable family fee relative to what is affordable for you.

I feel sure all doctors of chiropractic enjoy their practice most when caring for people who think healthy by trying to take some responsibility for their own health. This is one of the main objectives of the *Home Chiropractic Handbook*. Although the student will never have the experience of the doctor of chiropractic, through the understanding and application of this handbook, a finer rapport and appreciation in the doctor-patient relationship will develop.

In summary, common sense should dictate when to see a professional chiropractor. The principled chiropractor will clearly explain the chiropractic philosophy, and if spinal analysis indicates, will follow up with a specific scientific spinal adjustment that will release the power within that heals. He will further endeavor to bring out every positive aspect of his spinal analysis. You will recognize his adjustment given with confident hands and his voice will be firm and strong, suggesting the beneficial results he expects to see.

The following chapters elaborate on the life principle of

chiropractic. However, the ideas presented henceforth are not distinctly original with the chiropractic philosophy. They represent a greater understanding of how life expresses through the subconscious and conscious portions of the mind and manifests through the body. These chapters extend even deeper into the essential make up of man and reveal in greater detail other factors which contribute to a total health maintenance program for the entire family. I wish to pass on to you the appropriate ideas, combining words as best I can to convey to you that there is a great subconscious power within you now, awaiting your command. All you need do is study and apply the principle involved. It is my sincere hope that you will enjoy and benefit from the next two chapters most of all.

Chapter 9

The Educated Mind, The Innate Mind and the Life Principle of Chiropractic

To begin this chapter we will consult *Webster's Dictionary* concerning the word life: "an animating and shaping force or principle." The construction of the human body is without doubt the greatest and most complex form on earth. Every doctor who has diligently studied the anatomy and physiology of the human body is humbled by its magnificence in construction and performance. To illustrate clearly the magnificence of the life principle in the body, I offer the following example:

A person could choose to eat a peanut butter-jelly sandwich. He can put it into his mouth, chew it up and then swallow it. That is all he can do! Now the great subconscious power takes that peanut butter-jelly sandwich and converts it into blood, lymph, bone, muscle, skin, etc. In other words, it converts the sandwich into living tissue. The person's brain is made from that sandwich. While there are scientists who know what that sandwich is made of and how the nutrients are utilized in the body, there is no doctor, chemist, physicist or anyone that can create a single living cell out of peanut butter and jelly!

Yet still greater than the body itself is the *life* which flows through it shaping and stirring it to animation. This thing or stuff called life is what we want to discuss in this chapter. Our first premise must be to admit that we do not know what life is. No one knows what life is in its essence. But we can see that it is a force or power that flows and expresses through the various forms.

173

Even though man can never know what life is, *he can know how it expresses its power through the forms.* This is what I want to bring into focus for you in a precise and logical manner.

In the previous paragraphs we have postulated that life is an unknown power or principle animating the human form. We can further say that this life in the human form must be the same power flowing through all forms on earth. *Life in one form is the same as the life in all other variety of forms.* As an analogy, electricity in science is an unknown power. The scientist cannot tell you what electricity is, only how it works. Should you ask a scientist, "What is electricity?" he will give you a description of how it works, describing how it expresses through various man-made forms such as an electric toaster or radio, etc. Yet he will be unable to tell you what electricity is in its essence. There is only one power called electricity. In other words, there are not two electricities. The same electricity expresses through forms in varying degrees, from a small expression such as a simple electrical door bell up through higher forms such as a radio or television and on up through a complex computer. In all cases it is the same power called electricity making the forms function. *Likewise, there is just one life in all forms expressing varying degrees of consciousness and intelligence.* We need to understand how this life or unknown power functions through our form, as this is our right and privilege. I have already explained in previous chapters that the brain and spinal cord represent the master controlling system through which this power expresses. It is now opportune to show further how you can cooperate in harmony with the power or life in your form.

Now perhaps you have guessed what does the healing in the body. Why, of course, it is this unknown power! There are no doctors, no scientists, no human beings that have ever healed anything. None of them even know what life is! How could they heal anything! *The one power that created the body heals the body.* The job of doctors should simply be to get the parts in order so that the healing life power can express properly through the form. Your job will be to study this handbook and strive to correct spinal misalignments to keep life expressing in a healthy normal

174

manner, from brain cell to tissue cell. Ponder this fact deeply: the life power in older people is the same age as in a newborn baby. The body (which is the form) ages, not the life flowing through the form. Therefore, if we begin now in the human race to give proper health maintenance to the forms, then life would be like a candle burning just as bright, if not brighter, as the candle gets shorter, until finally the candle is so short that the flame sputters once or twice and goes out. The flame is the life and the candle is the form or body.

In explaining the educated mind and the innate mind, I offer this simple schematic drawing upon which I will elaborate. *This little stick man drawing should be taken very seriously as its simple description is profound and exact.* Just as man has discovered the laws of electricity, we also can discover the laws of living life in the body.

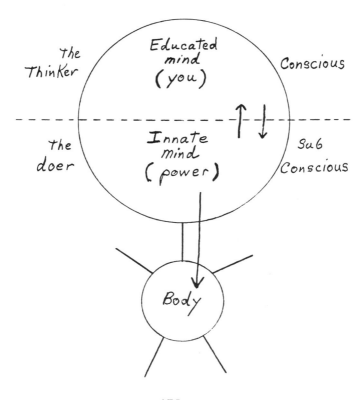

The brain has been divided into many areas for study and each area controls various functions in the body. However, this brain is such a complex computer that scientists have estimated that to duplicate one human brain, they would have to build a computer the size of the State of Texas and as high as the Empire State Building. So . . . we will keep the facts simple but exact with the stick man drawing.

You have two (2) parts to your mind. One is the conscious portion which is educated through school and experience. This is where you do your conscious thinking.

The second part that is much larger and more vast is the subconscious where the innate power within does all the work controlling your body.

It is this relationship between you (the "thinker") and the power (the "doer") that must be understood. *The word mind is just a name given to describe the activity of brain cells functioning between the conscious and subconscious portions of the physical brain.* If you went to a doctors' dissection laboratory and sliced the human brain of a cadaver, into microscopically thin slices, you would not find a physical thing or part called the mind. The mind is not a thing. *It is an activity.* As there has been much confusion regarding this, I offer the following example as proof of my statement:

As you are reading here, I will bring up a word. The word is *apple.* A few seconds ago you were not conscious of an apple, but now it has come up from the subconscious portion (where all your memory pictures and experiences are kept) to the conscious portion. Therefore, this action shows the activity of the thing we call the mind. The term mind is just a label.

In like manner, when we say that the sun rises or sets at a certain time, this is totally false, as the earth is constantly rotating on its axis and traveling around the sun. But for easy description we refer to the sun as rising and setting. Likewise, we will use the term mind for easy description of the activity between the educated, conscious portion and the innate subconscious portion. As you are looking at the stick man drawing, visualize that in the conscious portion, through your five physical senses: seeing,

176

hearing, smelling, tasting and touching; you are actually educating your mind. Impressions come to you through these five outer senses and your education in life is built around what comes to you in this way. All the interpretations of the five senses are done in your brain. In reality you actually see with your brain, hear with your brain, smell with your brain, taste with your brain, and touch with your brain. In other words, the five organs of sense are just the receivers of outside stimuli and the conscious educated brain is what first comes in contact with them for interpretation. Once the conscious portion has picked up an impression from the outside it relays it to the subconscious where it is recorded in memory for life. Just like the apple example given previously, is now stored in memory. I might say, "There is a fruit called a mango." If you have no picture come to your consciousness, you would have to investigate to see if there is such a fruit. If you could find a mango, your subconscious memory would always have a picture of that fruit.

Now how are all these facts related to health? Your ideas or concepts concerning health come to you via your senses. They are then programmed in memory in your great subconscious mind where all the power is. *The innate subconscious mind records every experience exactly as the educated conscious mind interprets it, true or false, good or bad.* Some of your concepts concerning health may have been false and yet without investigation you could have accepted them as truth, such as the idea of germs causing disease. You will have to investigate this concept.

Perhaps this handbook has been filled with new ideas for you, in which case you will have to investigate each one and reason upon it. If upon reasoning you can prove they are factual, then you have a truth. A fact is something that can be proved to yourself or one to another.

Reason implies that you have a choice to believe or disbelieve what has been presented. However, by reasoning through logic to a fact is to discover a truth. For example, there may have been a time when you believed in Santa Claus, which was fine for a little mind. But through *logical reasoning,* you came to the fact that there isn't any man called Santa living at the North Pole and thus

177

you have a truth fixed in your subconscious computer forever.

So you can see that the conscious educated mind can reason and choose true concepts or false concepts, positive ideas or negative ideas, depending on how well you think ideas out using logic. *The subconscious mind has all the power. It is the doer* and carries out the order or suggestion in your body or environment. Perhaps this is what the great teacher meant when he said, "As a man thinketh in his heart so is he." You become what you program your great subconscious computer to perform in your life.

The subconscious computer can be reprogrammed from fantasy to fact just like the "Santa story." The trouble has been that people still believe the fantasy as truth, such as believing that doctors heal. If you can accept, through *logical reasoning,* that it is not the doctor that does the healing but the power within the body which built the body that does the healing, then you are on the right track to solving health problems. You can then go to any type of doctor *if necessary* and accept his pills, treatments, and adjustments knowing that with the right concept placed into the great subconscious, you will regain health. Of course the idea or concept of correcting the spine is a most logical approach to health maintenance and can be considered a fact in caring for the physical body. However, it would be illogical to state that vertebral misalignments are the only cause of disease in the body. Other factors must be considered in order to enter a total health picture. These will be discussed in the final chapter. At this point, you have a way to obtain much health through spinal correcting. And by understanding how the educated and innate mind works, you can see what takes over and does the healing after you correct a vertebra into its proper position. In leading you into the next chapter, we have stated that vertebral misalignments cause disease in the body and by correcting them you are correcting a cause and not treating an effect. The last question to ask would naturally be, "What are the causes of vertebral misalignments and what other factors contribute to total health?"

Chapter 10
Four Essential Body Requirements and The Effect of Positive or Negative Emotions

In the first eight chapters of this handbook we have thoroughly considered a major aspect of physical health: a healthy unimpaired transmission of life energy from brain cell to tissue cell. We have shown conclusively that the brain and spinal cord is the master controlling system of each of the six major systems of the body. We have presented fundamentals of anatomy to acquaint you with this relationship. We have further given you a way to apply the knowledge practically by correcting misalignments in your own home.

In Chapter Nine we began a new topic that intimately related the life principle in expression through the educated and innate portions of the mind. This chapter will take this idea a step further and correlate this life principle with the man who lives inside the body. It will show conclusively through logical reason *that the body is just one big effect of what the man who lives inside wills the body to be.*

When a person pays respect to the deceased at a funeral, he may stand there looking at the person, but what he is really looking at is the person's body. The person who lived inside the body is gone. Again life is an unknown. Reasoning to a logical conclusion, when life left that body, so did the man who lived inside. Therefore, the fact that you are reading this book and seeing these words with your eyes and analyzing these ideas in your

179

educated brain indicates that you are inside that form we call the human body.

In the last scientific analysis, the body is understood to be just so much matter put together in a very wonderful way. But without the person living inside operating the body, it will quickly return to dust. You might think of your body as your instrument with which you perform your tasks.

Therefore, it is of utmost importance that you understand the relationship between you and the power or life in the body.

It is now postulated by modern medical science that 80 to 90 percent of all disease is caused by stress. Let's analyze stress and determine exactly what causes it and how it affects our health.

If we observe ourselves responding to outside stimuli in a negative way, without the use of logical reasoning, we will generally react to what comes our way via the five senses, in an emotionally disturbed manner. This reactionary behavior upsets our master controlling computer (brain and spinal cord) which in turn upsets the other six major systems and ultimately affects the entire body in a deleterious way. Under stress, we find hormonal activities accelerated resulting in an imbalance of the glandular system; in the eliminative system stress may result in constipation or excessive excretions; the nerve system becomes one that is nervous, impairing healthy nerve transmission; all normal digestive processes — absorption, distribution, assimilation, and elimination — are inhibited; muscles tend to tighten and even become strained as a result of stress; the circulatory system is affected by an increase in heartrate, and constriction of the blood vessels causing a rise in blood pressure. *Therefore, stress can be summed up as the inability of a person to successfully adapt to the environment.*

Fight or flight responses to outside stimuli may have been appropriate behavior during a previous era. However, in modern society we repress the natural expression of these tendencies and therefore cause stress and disease in the body. Today there is no logical reason for man to fight or flee most situations in life. In all but life-threatening situations man must first:

1) hold any emotional reaction in check;

180

2) apply logical reason as to whether you can change the situation, or adapt to it, if it is not within your power to change.

In these two ways one can accept most situations appearing as negative, by changing them or adapting to them, and thus peace and balance can be maintained in the body and environment. Therefore, instead of reacting to or repressing undesirable situations (stimuli) the individual can endeavor to *act* in an intelligent manner according to what each new problem demands. This can be accomplished by applying logical reason to every situation life presents.

Negative emotions cause stress in the body and stress causes disease. To give you an idea of what negative emotions are I shall list a few and then explain how they are the cause of disease and the disturbed body is the effect. Fear, worry, anger, jealousy, destructive criticism, hypocrisy and hate are some of the negative emotions that one can express in the conscious educated mind. Further, with repetition they can be driven down into the subconscious innate mind where they will actually become fixed as stressful behavior patterns that continually disturb normal body functions.

When an individual expresses, for instance, anger and jealousy, the entire human body is affected adversely, not to mention the negativity he sends forth into the environment. Anger and jealousy actually begin interfering with the brain's messages to body parts. His muscles are always tense, most often in the neck and back. Because muscles attach to bones, muscle tension causes an uneven pulling and ultimately misaligns vertebrae. Thus organic breakdown of the body begins due to lack of normal nerve transmission, brain cell to tissue cell. An example can be given of a man coming to my office complaining of headaches and stomach ulcers. I could examine his spine and undoubtedly find subluxations in the cervical and thoracic regions limiting nerve transmission to the stomach and head. I could adjust these vertebral misalignments, but if the man is constantly expressing any negative emotions such as the ones we are discussing — anger and Jealousy — then I would simply be adjusting the effect. His

181

vertebrae will again become misaligned in a short time due to the stress caused by these negative emotions, and his body will continue downhill to serious disease. Likewise, he can see any type of doctor in search for health and each doctor will treat the effect by altering the body in some way. The cause is the incorrect programming of his subconscious computer. He must seek a doctor that can find the cause behind the effect, or he must discover it for himself. In summary of the negative emotions, it can be stated that these types of emotions create turmoil in the body, resulting in disease and further culminate in unhappiness and confusion.

On the opposite side of the emotional scale, we have the positive emotions such as faith, hope, patience, courage, kindness, and love. These emotions are also our choice to make consciously. When a person is involved in these positive emotions on a continual basis, his body is free from stress, and he is more apt to experience normal health. *Positive emotions can build health and happiness bringing peace to the individual expressing them providing that the individual has balanced his thinking.*

People who have tried "positive thinking" often set up a polarity (an extreme) of only good in their minds, and this gets them emotionally high. They will attract others to them who are in need of help or encouragement. Inevitably they will be dragged down into the negativity of the person asking for positive encouragement. At this point they become convinced that positive thinking does not work and will revert back to their negative way of thinking.

To further recognize the effects of positive and negative emotions it must be understood that both are opposites. Positive and negative are the opposites of each other. Since many people have cultivated the negative and created stress and ultimately disease, it becomes necessary to cultivate the positive, as the positive will create a more desirable condition. One might say the scale has been tipped to negative and must now have positive added to the opposite end. The key is to balance the scale, not tip it completely to the positive. This can be done by understanding your emotions and then controlling them!

182

If the emotions are properly controlled, one could choose to express anger in a constructive way without becoming entangled in the emotion itself. For clarification I offer the following example. A child who requires reprimand may need to observe his parents showing anger as he is being disciplined in order that the discipline be effective. If the parent is reasoning logically he will know that all children require discipline at times and therefore there is no reason for the parent to actually be angry and upset. The parent should simply take appropriate action that is necessary and not become emotionally angry. *The key to expressing the positive is to balance your thinking by controlling your emotions, both negative and positive.* With control the individual will not become off-balanced on the emotion itself. Rather, the person will be able to express emotions in a manner that is appropriate for each circumstance life presents.

I would like to continue by discussing the art and power of suggestion and its relationship in producing health and happiness. As a fact, everything you see, hear, smell, taste, and touch is a suggestion that comes into your conscious, educated mind and is then impressed in the subconscious, innate mind. It becomes of paramount importance then, that you stay on guard as to what suggestions you allow to strongly impress the subconscious.

If you convey to a child over and over again that he is stupid, dumb, or that he is sickly or looks sickly, these suggestions impress his little educated mind and very quickly pass down into the child's subconscious innate mind. I use the word "quickly" because the child does not have the intellectual capacity to doubt or question a person whom he loves and respects as an authority. If the suggestion is repeated, it will become a powerful subconscious influence in the child's life and will surely manifest in the child's body or environment. Always suggest to children and everyone constructive, healthful suggestions. Say, "You can do it," "You can get better," "You can get well," "You can learn," etc. Doctors are usually reluctant to tell patients that they will get well simply because they fear a lawsuit if the patient does not recover. If the suggestion is not repeated over and over and if the patient will not accept the beneficial suggestion, then the doctor is not to blame.

Some people consciously, with their educated minds, block out and will not accept good, healthy constructive ideas. They actually choose to think sick, unhealthy thoughts. Until these people learn to reason correctly and become aware that they can actually direct the great power in the subconscious mind, they will always be sick and unhappy.

With your family members practice giving healthy, happy constructive suggestions to each other. Practice on yourself as well by giving your own subconscious innate mind constructive suggestions. As you develop confidence that suggestion really works just as shown on the stick man diagram, then you can be absolutely affirmative and say, "I will," "I will get well," "I will be healthy," etc. Suggest these and any other constructive ideas you wish to manifest to your own subconscious. Repetition is a key to success in practicing the art of suggestion, just as it was required for mastery of the multiplication tables.

Another key to manifesting constructive ideas through suggestion is to visualize the result. See what you want as though it has already happened, and this will further impress the great subconscious innate power with the desired result. Most people use this in the negative way. They may suggest the positive constructive idea but then visualize the opposite and thus confuse their mind. So to keep it straight: suggest what you want and then visualize it by using your imaginative faculty to see it as though it has come to be.

When giving a spinal correction to a family member, always suggest with the physical correcting technique the positive result you expect to see manifest. Giving a good suggestion to another is an art. By this I mean the suggestion will not be effective, especially in an adult, if it is given in a "wishy-washy," half-confident manner. Give the suggestion with a firm and authoritative voice visualizing the result as though it has come to be.

So dear friend, choose ideas that are positive and constructive and let only those enter deep into the subconscious innate mind. The power therein will carry out the idea it has received. It may take some time according to the breadth of the idea and suggestion, but if you persist with determination to succeed, *you will succeed.* Your body will be healthy and you will be happier and by example, able to show others how to take charge of their lives so they may find health and happiness.

What I have presented regarding how suggestion works through the conscious educated mind and into the subconscious innate power is an exact law. As an analogy, if a farmer sows corn seed into his field, with proper care, he will harvest corn. The farmer would not plant wheat seed and expect to reap corn. Likewise if you expect to reap health and happiness, *you must plant seeds of health and happiness in your subconscious garden.* You must continue to nurture your planted seeds with a full scope of happy, healthful ideas. These ideas must conform to your logical reason. In other words, you cannot plant health ideas in your subconscious and then go merrily along disobeying the four body requirements (the four essential body requirements will be explained in the remainder of this chapter).

To get you on your way in establishing total health and much greater peace and happiness, I offer the following criteria in orderly sequence, for your consideration.

1. If your body has been in poor health, correct the physical problem through spinal correcting or see a doctor *if necessary;*
2. *Immediately* resolve to choose the positive and express your emotions constructively as this will help balance your thinking;
3. Begin planting seeds (ideas) of health and happiness in your subconscious garden;
4. Take action to begin obeying the four essential body requirements;
5. Most important, apply your inner faculties of *will* and *imagination* by using *repetition* and *visualization.* Actually picture how you will look and feel once you are happy and healthy.

If emotional and health problems have been serious, it may take a little more time to manifest the result you desire. Diligently apply these last five steps in your life and *you can be assured of experiencing greater health and happiness.*

The four essential requirements of the body that are part of the title of this chapter will now be briefly discussed. The word essential is used to describe the body requirements because each one must be understood and provided for the body.

First is the body requirement of *nourishment*. Much has been written on nourishment and most of the literature on nourishment tends to confuse rather than simplify. In grammar school we were taught the names of various foods; however, these foods were improperly categorized. It is my intention to simply explain how, why, and in what way the body needs to be nourished. There are four classes of foods; namely,

1. "builders"
2. "eliminators"
3. "sweets and starches"
4. "lubricators."

Before I begin explaining the essential body requirement of nourishment, it is necessary that you understand what is meant by "dead" devitalized food and "live" food. Dead foods have been preserved, cooked and tampered with, destroying some or all of the original vitamins and enzymes. Dead food can be considered as any food that is not in its natural state. On the other hand, live foods are those that nature has grown and come to us in their natural state. More will be said concerning live foods in the presentation of the eliminative class of foods.

The first class called the "builders" is named as such because they build the body. However, they all form acid and most people should eat only one builder food per meal. Examples of builder foods include: all dairy products, eggs, all meat, fish, fowl, kidney beans, lima beans, navy beans, and all nuts. The builder foods simply build the body.

The second class of food is the "eliminators." This type of food breaks down old dead cells in the body and repairs damaged tissue, ridding the body of waste material. Eliminators are the major key in nutrition that can assure the body of replacing old worn out cells with new healthy cells. Although preserved fruits and vegetables (without added sugar) are eliminative food, raw fruits and vegetables are alive. In a natural, raw state these provide the most complete range of vitamins, minerals and other nutrients as well as living substance. Therefore, these are the best source of eliminative food. Daily intake of eliminative food should always include raw natural fruits and vegetables. To have a properly functioning eliminative system, everyone should eat as much eliminative food as builder food, per meal. Fresh squeezed lemon juice is a most powerful eliminative food. Fresh squeezed lemon juice and warm water is highly recommended if a person's body resistance has been low and in need of revitalization. Other eliminative foods are limes, grapefruits, oranges, peaches, apricots, apples, plums, pears, cherries, tomatoes, currents, all berries, all melons, pineapple, and all fruit except bananas . Also included under eliminative foods are the following vegetables: spinach, carrots, celery, parsley, lettuce, green peppers, Swiss chard, onions, cucumbers, cabbage, cauliflower, peas and string beans, beets, endive, asparagus, dandelion, artichokes, summer squash, kale, broccoli, watercress, and all other vegetables except potatoes, avocadoes, dried peas and dried beans. Potatoes, dried peas and dried beans are not eliminative foods as they contain starch. Avocadoes contain fat and protein. If you cook your vegetables in water, drink the broth as it contains much of the mineral content of the vegetables. Once you become accustomed to eating as much eliminative food as builder food you will be surprised how healthy your body has become.

The *third class* of foods are sweets and starches. The purpose of these types of foods is to keep oxygen soluble with minerals for the release of energy in the body. As whole grains are the most complete source of B-complex vitamins, a sufficient amount should be taken in daily. Whole grains will also provide fiber to help maintain normal bowel elimination. Sweets should supplement the daily diet only if extra calories are needed. Make note sweets and starches can cause congestion in the body if too much is eaten. Sweets are: bananas, honey, sugar, molasses, candy, soft drinks, all dried fruit, any food containing sugar. Starches are: flour, cereals, dried corn, all breads, macaroni, spaghetti, noodles, all potatoes, and grains made into flour and cereals.

The *fourth class* of foods are called the "lubricators." Their primary purpose is to lubricate the body; however, some of them also build the body. This class of foods include butter, vegetable oils, olive oil, avocadoes, and all fats. A thin person may eat as much of this type as desired. However, a person that is too heavy should eat a minimal amount of lubricator foods.

With regard to drinking, everyone should drink water each day, at least three glasses. Considering the body is approximately 95 percent water, it is essential to flush the body with clean water each day. However, water does not cleanse the body. *Fruits and vegetables in the eliminator class cleanse the body,* and this is the reason everyone needs to eat as much eliminative food as builder food.

The four classes of foods I have presented are simply outlined in regard to the way they are utilized in the body. Nourishing your body properly does not have to be complicated the way most all nutrition and diet books on the market today make it seem. Reread these classes and then prepare meals so that you receive the following amount of each class, in this order:

1. one type of builder per meal
2. one or more varieties of eliminators per meal
3. if still hungry, eat sweets and starches (especially whole grains)
4. lubricators as needed

While everyone needs to comply with the essential body requirement of nourishment, it must be accomplished with regard to the needs of each individual. For example, if you are engaged in a physically demanding job, you may need to take in a little more of the sweets and starches and builder foods. However, always include a proportionate amount of eliminative food to maintain good health.

Do not force yourself to eat. Eat only when you naturally feel hungry. If you are obeying the requirement of exercise, then sooner or later you will naturally develop an appetite.

The second essential body requirement is *exercise.* All body muscles and joints must be moved each day. In order to absorb and distribute the nourishment required by the body, the cir-

188

culatory system must be stimulated. However, it is not recommended that you employ a regemented set of exercises outlined by someone who is unfamiliar with your individual needs. Choose sports or exercises that you naturally enjoy. In so doing it will be easy and pleasurable to comply with this requirement without much discipline. Everyone on this earth is an individual with a unique body build and therefore should choose sports and exercises to suit his particular body type and frame. Do not let someone or some book con you into a system of exercises unless it naturally appeals to you! Yet remember, that this requirement of exercise must be fulfilled in order that the circulatory system perform its normal functions of absorption, distribution, assimilation and elimination. Moving all muscles and joints each day is the only way to stimulate the circulatory system. When engaging in your chosen sport or exercise, the muscles will naturally become tired relative to their tonus and condition. This feeling of tiredness is your indication that you have worked your body enough.

Oftentimes in the logging community where I practice, logger patients will finish work in the woods late and come into my office exceedingly tired in need of a chiropractic spinal adjustment. With eyes half opened they will frequently ask me, "Do you think I should take some kind of exercise, Doc?" I ask them, "Are you tired when you get home from work?" They will answer, "When I've been working real hard, I can hardly stay awake to eat my supper." When I explain that it is obvious that their bodies have had enough exercise for the day, they always laugh and say, "Yeh, you're right," then go home for some recuperation.

The third essential requirement of the body is *recuperation.* This requirement demands that every human being must have sufficient rest and sleep. Every body needs time to recuperate and to repair. However, the body requirement of recupration does not mean sleep only. There are three aspects of recuperation which are listed as follows:

1. Sleep
2. Rest
3. Recreation

Everyone needs sufficient sleep relative to his lifestyle. Each person needs physical rest and mental rest. One needs to provide time each day to relax the body and as well to collect his thoughts in a quiet surrounding. Simply relax and let go of the day's activities and enjoy this time. The last aspect of recuperation is recreation. We must all play, laugh and have fun. Set aside time on a regular basis for you and your family to play and have fun. Find something each member of the family enjoys. Hobbies and recreational activities provide opportunities to develop inherent talents and abilities in a way that work or school life does not always allow. Through recreation the brain enjoys a change of pace. Different brain cells are stimulated in play and laughter. This allows the cells of the brain that are active in work, to have time to rest. *This combination of play and laughter and recreation followed by rest will assure sound sleep and help maintain health in the body and mind.*

The fourth and last essential requirement of the body is *sanitation*. To most people sanitation means keeping the outside of the body clean. This is only one aspect of sanitation. The second aspect is to keep the inside of the body clean. This is accomplished by drinking plenty of water each day and more importantly the body must have plenty of fruits and vegetables everyday. As stated before at least an equal amount of eliminative food to builder food will assure a clean body inside, providing one also receives proper exercise for his individual body type. To further cleanse the body a person should exercise enough to induce perspiration which naturally eliminates waste material from the body through the pores of the skin. If one has properly nourished his body and has intelligently exercised to stimulate the circulatory system and further provides proper recuperation so that all body systems can rejuvenate, then inner-body sanitation is naturally and easily maintained. This concludes my explanation of the four essential requirements of the body.

In bringing this book to a close I would like to say that I have only briefly touched upon the idea of total health and happiness in the last two chapters. *There is a way* for you to obtain health, happiness and peace. Considering the Creator built such a magnificent and beautiful body for us to live in, it is no less than

190

our duty to learn the laws of the body and further learn the laws relating to the man or woman living inside the body. In this way you will be able to choose and express constructive ideas that bring health, happiness and peace.

A complete and thorough explanation of the last two chapters in this handbook is offered in a book called *Rays of the Dawn* and the *Concept-Therapy Philosophy*, both originated and written by Dr. Thurman Fleet in 1931.

The book *Rays of the Dawn* is available for purchase as well as free literature and information by contacting:

The Concept-Therapy Institute
25550 Boerne Stage Road
San Antonio, Texas 78255-9565
(512) 698-2254
or call
TOLL FREE
1-800-531-5628

The book that I bring to your attention, called *Rays of the Dawn,* I believe to be the greatest piece of literature ever written in the history of modern man. In conclusion I hope you have enjoyed and will study and apply the *Home Chiropractic Handbook* and soon obtain a copy of *Rays of the Dawn* by Dr. Thurman Fleet.

My best to you,

Dr. Karl V. Holmquist

Photography Acknowledgment

The original color photographs for this handbook were taken by:

Dwain Mason's Studio of Fine Photography
725 Murdock
Sedro Woolley, Washington 98284

When I conveyed to Dwain Mason what type of photographic presentation I needed, he was able to take each and every photo perfect on the first click of his camera. I thank Dwain Mason for his expertise in fine photography.

Editing Acknowledgment

I gratefully thank my wife, E. Renee Holmquist, B.A., M.S., for her most helpful editing, as well as Charlie Roberts and Burleigh Jones for their long hours of diligent assistance in preparing this manuscript.

Acknowledgment of References

I would like to individually acknowledge the following books for the information I have received. However, in writing this handbook, there have been absolutely no direct quotes, phrases or paragraphs taken from any of the following books.

The two anatomy textbooks used for reference to compile my freehand drawings are *Gray's Anatomy* and *Chiropractic Orthopedy*. *Chiropractic Orthopedy* is appreciated for its excellent descriptions of spinal anatomy. *Gray's Anatomy* is appreciated for its excellent descriptions of complete human anatomy.

Webster's Seventh New Collegiate Dictionary has provided unbiased definitions relating to many topics in this handbook.

I would like to acknowledge the courage of Dr. Robert S. Mendelsohn, M.D., in writing *Confessions of a Medical Heretic.*

The knowledge gleaned from the study of the *Rays of the Dawn, Concept-Therapy* text, and the texts of all seven phases of Conceptology has been most illuminating. Above all, the author of this handbook wishes to acknowledge his great indebtedness for the wisdom received through the Concept-Therapy Philosophy.